THE ITALIAN I

FOR ATHLETES *Cookbook*

The Best 220+ Seafood and Vegetarian Recipes
for Weight Loss and Heart Health!
Stay FIT and LIGHT with The Most
Delicious Diet Overall!

2 BOOKS IN 1

By

Olivia Rossi

Table of Contents

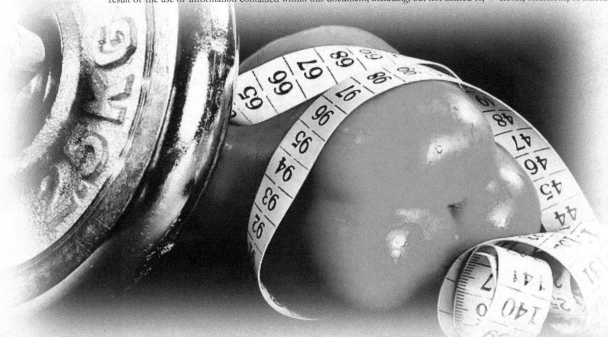

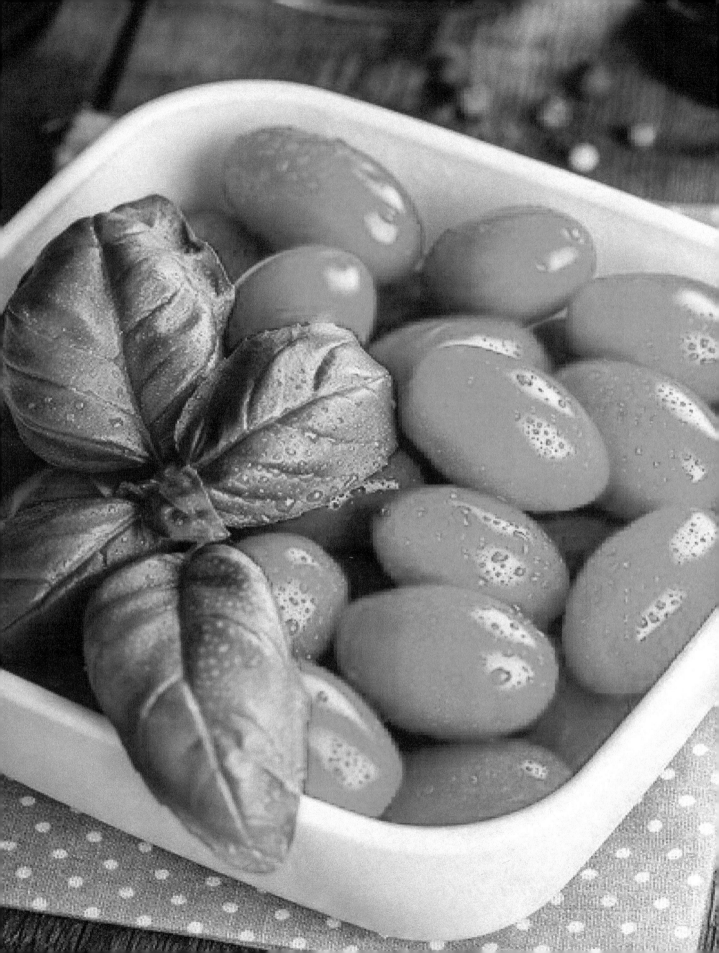

Introduction

Have you ever eaten Italian dishes?

Italian Cuisine is one of the most delicious in all of the world!

Italian Cuisine is also one of the HEALTHIEST diets overall!

For this reason, everybody can follow Italian Diet: **children**, **older people**, **beginners**, **women**, and **men**! In my opinion, each man and woman, who want to stay FIT, should follow this diet absolutely: indeed, the Italian diet is perfect for weight loss and maintaining the body FIT and HEALTHY!

This is why I wanted to create this fantastic cookbook: "The Italian Diet for Athletes Cookbook" is the collection of "The Italian Diet for Men Cookbook" and "The Italian Diet for Women Cookbook", to give to my readers the best recipes for Heart Health and for having the Perfect Body! Italian cuisine is but a real... lifestyle!

Do you want to have a FIT and EERGETIC Body?

"The Italian Diet for Athletes Cookbook" is what you need!

What can you eat in Italian Cuisine?

- Cereals: bread, pasta, pizza
- Legumes: green beans, chickpeas, beans
- Proteins: milk, cheese, red meat, fish, light meat, seafood, nuts, extra virgin olive oil
- Fibers and vitamins: all of vegetables and fruits

Add raw extra virgin olive oil to your food for the best experience ever!

In the Italian Diet, it is important the quality of foods: foods must be fresh and, if possible, must be cultivated in Italy.

Do you want to know The Best 220 Italian Recipes for Athletes?

So, LET'S GO together!

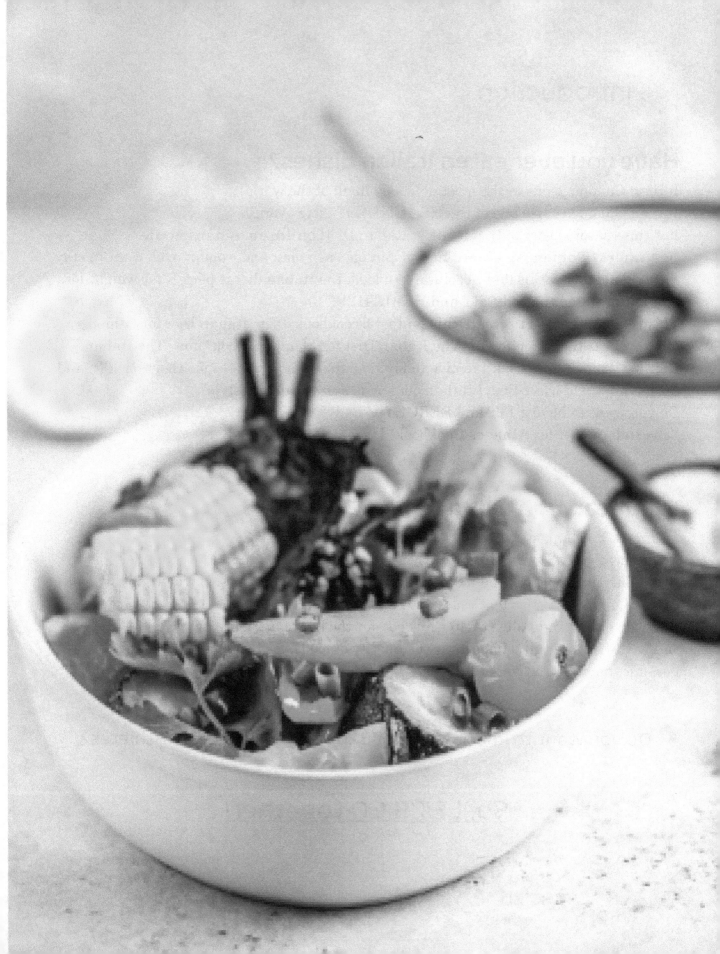

Chapter 1. BREAKFAST AND SNACKS

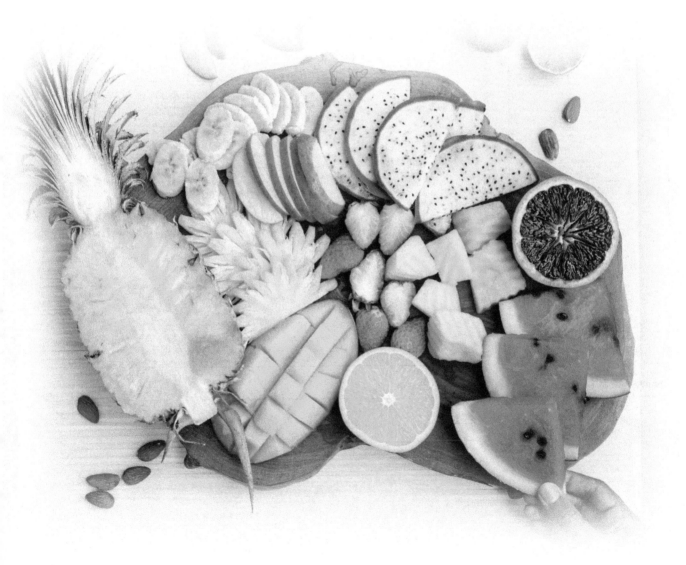

1) SPECIAL CAULIFLOWER FRITTERS AND HUMMUS

Cooking Time: 15 Minutes		Servings: 4

Ingredients:

- ✓ 2 (15 oz) cans chickpeas, divided
- ✓ 2 1/2 tbsp olive oil, divided, plus more for frying
- ✓ 1 cup onion, chopped, about 1/2 a small onion
- ✓ 2 tbsp garlic, minced
- ✓ 2 cups cauliflower, cut into small pieces, about 1/2 a large head
- ✓ 1/2 tsp salt
- ✓ black pepper
- ✓ Topping:
- ✓ Hummus, of choice
- ✓ Green onion, diced

Directions:

- ❖ Preheat oven to 400°F
- ❖ Rinse and drain 1 can of the chickpeas, place them on a paper towel to dry off well
- ❖ Then place the chickpeas into a large bowl, removing the loose skins that come off, and toss with 1 tbsp of olive oil, spread the chickpeas onto a large pan (being careful not to over-crowd them) and sprinkle with salt and pepper
- ❖ Bake for 20 minutes, then stir, and then bake an additional 5-10 minutes until very crispy
- ❖ Once the chickpeas are roasted, transfer them to a large food processor and process until broken down and crumble - Don't over process them and turn it into flour, as you need to have some texture. Place the mixture into a small bowl, set aside
- ❖ In a large pan over medium-high heat, add the remaining 1 1/2 tbsp of olive oil
- ❖ Once heated, add in the onion and garlic, cook until lightly golden brown, about 2 minutes. Then add in the chopped cauliflower, cook for an additional 2 minutes, until the cauliflower is golden
- ❖ Turn the heat down to low and cover the pan, cook until the cauliflower is fork tender and the onions are golden brown and caramelized, stirring often, about 3-5 minutes
- ❖ Transfer the cauliflower mixture to the food processor, drain and rinse the remaining can of chickpeas and add them into the food processor, along with the salt and a pinch of pepper. Blend until smooth, and the mixture starts to ball, stop to scrape down the sides as needed
- ❖ Transfer the cauliflower mixture into a large bowl and add in 1/2 cup of the roasted chickpea crumbs (you won't use all of the crumbs, but it is easier to break them down when you have a larger amount.), stir until well combined
- ❖ In a large bowl over medium heat, add in enough oil to lightly cover the bottom of a large pan
- ❖ Working in batches, cook the patties until golden brown, about 2-3 minutes, flip and cook again
- ❖ Distribute among the container, placing parchment paper in between the fritters. Store in the fridge for 2-3 days
- ❖ To Serve: Heat through in the oven at 350F for 5-8 minutes. Top with hummus, green onion and enjoy!
- ❖ Recipe Notes: Don't add too much oil while frying the fritter or they will end up soggy. Use only enough to cover the pan. Use a fork while frying and resist the urge to flip them every minute to see if they are golden

Nutrition: Calories:333;Total Carbohydrates: 45g;Total Fat: 13g;Protein: 14g

2) ITALIAN BREAKFAST SAUSAGE AND NEW POTATOES WITH VEGETABLES

	Cooking Time: 30 Minutes	Servings: 4

✓ 1 lbs sweet Italian sausage links, sliced on the bias (diagonal) ✓ 2 cups baby potatoes, halved ✓ 2 cups broccoli florets ✓ 1 cup onions cut to 1-inch chunks ✓ 2 cups small mushrooms -half or quarter the large ones for uniform size	✓ 1 cup baby carrots ✓ 2 tbsp olive oil ✓ 1/2 tsp garlic powder ✓ 1/2 tsp Italian seasoning ✓ 1 tsp salt ✓ 1/2 tsp pepper	❖ Preheat the oven to 400 degrees F ❖ In a large bowl, add the baby potatoes, broccoli florets, onions, small mushrooms, and baby carrots ❖ Add in the olive oil, salt, pepper, garlic powder and Italian seasoning and toss to evenly coat ❖ Spread the vegetables onto a sheet pan in one even layer ❖ Arrange the sausage slices on the pan over the vegetables ❖ Bake for 30 minutes – make sure to sake halfway through to prevent sticking ❖ Allow to cool ❖ Distribute the Italian sausages and vegetables among the containers and store in the fridge for 2-3 days ❖ To Serve: Reheat in the microwave for 1-2 minutes, or until heated through and enjoy! ❖ Recipe Notes: If you would like crispier potatoes, place them on the pan and bake for 15 minutes before adding the other ingredients to the pan.

3) GREEK QUINOA BREAKFAST BOWL

	Cooking Time: 20 Minutes	Servings: 6

✓ 12 eggs ✓ ¼ cup plain Greek yogurt ✓ 1 tsp onion powder ✓ 1 tsp granulated garlic ✓ ½ tsp salt ✓ ½ tsp pepper	✓ 1 tsp olive oil ✓ 1 (5 oz) bag baby spinach ✓ 1 pint cherry tomatoes, halved ✓ 1 cup feta cheese ✓ 2 cups cooked quinoa	❖ In a large bowl whisk together eggs, Greek yogurt, onion powder, granulated garlic, salt, and pepper, set aside ❖ In a large skillet, heat olive oil and add spinach, cook the spinach until it is slightly wilted, about 3-4 minutes. Add in cherry tomatoes, cook until tomatoes are softened, 4 minutes. Stir in egg mixture and cook until the eggs are set, about 7-9 minutes, stir in the eggs as they cook to scramble ❖ Once the eggs have set stir in the feta and quinoa, cook until heated through. Distribute evenly among the containers, store for 2-3 days ❖ To serve: Reheat in the microwave for 30 seconds to 1 minute or heated through

4) EGG, HAM AND CHEESE SANDWICHES IN THE FREEZER

	Cooking Time: 20 Minutes	Servings: 6

✓ Cooking spray or oil to grease the baking dish ✓ 7 large eggs ✓ ½ cup low-fat (2%) milk ✓ ½ tsp garlic powder ✓ ½ tsp onion powder	✓ 1 tbsp Dijon mustard ✓ ½ tsp honey ✓ 6 whole-wheat English muffins ✓ 6 slices thinly sliced prosciutto ✓ 6 slices Swiss cheese	❖ Preheat the oven to 375°F. Lightly oil or spray an 8-by--inch glass or ceramic baking dish with cooking spray. ❖ In a large bowl, whisk together the eggs, milk, garlic powder, and onion powder. Pour the mixture into the baking dish and bake for minutes, until the eggs are set and no longer jiggling. Cool. ❖ While the eggs are baking, mix the mustard and honey in a small bowl. Lay out the English muffin halves to start assembly. ❖ When the eggs are cool, use a biscuit cutter or drinking glass about the same size as the English muffin diameter to cut 6 egg circles. Divide the leftover egg scraps evenly to be added to each sandwich. ❖ Spread ½ tsp of honey mustard on each of the bottom English muffin halves. Top each with 1 slice of prosciutto, 1 egg circle and scraps, 1 slice of cheese, and the top half of the muffin. ❖ Wrap each sandwich tightly in foil. ❖

5) HEALTHY SALAD ZUCCHINI CABBAGE TOMATO

	Cooking Time: 20 Minutes	**Servings:** 4

Ingredients:

- ✓ 1 lb kale, chopped
- ✓ 2 tbsp fresh parsley, chopped
- ✓ 1 tbsp vinegar
- ✓ 1/2 cup can tomato, crushed
- ✓ 1 tsp paprika
- ✓ 1 cup zucchini, cut into cubes
- ✓ 1 cup grape tomatoes, halved
- ✓ 2 tbsp olive oil
- ✓ 1 onion, chopped
- ✓ 1 leek, sliced
- ✓ Pepper
- ✓ Salt

Directions:

- ❖ Add oil into the inner pot of instant pot and set the pot on sauté mode.
- ❖ Add leek and onion and sauté for 5 minutes.
- ❖ Add kale and remaining ingredients and stir well.
- ❖ Seal pot with lid and cook on high for 15 minutes.
- ❖ Once done, allow to release pressure naturally for 10 minutes then release remaining using quick release. Remove lid.
- ❖ Stir and serve.

Nutrition: Calories: 162;Fat: 3 g;Carbohydrates: 22.2 g;Sugar: 4.8 g;Protein: 5.2 g;Cholesterol: 0 mg

6) Bacon Brie omelette with radish salad

	Cooking Time: 10 Minutes	**Servings:** 6

Ingredients:

- ✓ 200 g smoked lardons
- ✓ 3 tsp olive oil, divided
- ✓ 7 ounces smoked bacon
- ✓ 6 lightly beaten eggs
- ✓ small bunch chives, snipped up
- ✓ 3½ ounces sliced brie
- ✓ 1 tsp red wine vinegar
- ✓ 1 tsp Dijon mustard
- ✓ 1 cucumber, deseeded, halved, and sliced up diagonally
- ✓ 7 ounces radish, quartered

Directions:

- ❖ Heat up the grill.
- ❖ Add 1 tsp of oil to a small pan and heat on the grill.
- ❖ Add lardons and fry them until nice and crisp.
- ❖ Drain the lardon on kitchen paper.
- ❖ Heat the remaining 2 tsp of oil in a non-sticking pan on the grill.
- ❖ Add lardons, eggs, chives, and ground pepper, and cook over low heat until semi-set.
- ❖ Carefully lay the Brie on top, and grill until it has set and is golden in color.
- ❖ Remove from pan and cut into wedges.
- ❖ Make the salad by mixing olive oil, mustard, vinegar, and seasoning in a bowl.
- ❖ Add cucumber and radish and mix well.
- ❖ Serve the salad alongside the Omelette wedges in containers.
- ❖ Enjoy!

7) OATMEAL WITH CRANBERRIES

	Cooking Time: 6 Minutes	**Servings:** 2

- ✓ 1/2 cup steel-cut oats
- ✓ 1 cup unsweetened almond milk
- ✓ 1 1/2 tbsp maple syrup
- ✓ 1/4 tsp cinnamon
- ✓ 1/4 tsp vanilla
- ✓ 1/4 cup dried cranberries
- ✓ 1 cup of water
- ✓ 1 tsp lemon zest, grated
- ✓ 1/4 cup orange juice

Directions:

- ❖ Add all ingredients into the heat-safe dish and stir well.
- ❖ Pour 1 cup of water into the instant pot then place the trivet in the pot.
- ❖ Place dish on top of the trivet.
- ❖ Seal pot with lid and cook on high for 6 minutes.
- ❖ Once done, allow to release pressure naturally for 10 minutes then release remaining using quick release. Remove lid.
- ❖ Serve and enjoy.

Nutrition: Calories: 161;Fat: 3.2 g;Carbohydrates: 29.9 g;Sugar: 12.4 g;Protein: 3.4 g;Cholesterol: 0 mg

8) FIGS TOAST WITH RICOTTA CHEESE

	Cooking Time: 15 Minutes	Servings: 1

Ingredients:

- ✓ 2 slices whole-wheat toast
- ✓ 1 tsp honey
- ✓ ¼ cup ricotta (partly skimmed)
- ✓ 1 dash cinnamon
- ✓ 2 figs (sliced)
- ✓ 1 tsp sesame seeds

Directions:

- ❖ Start by mixing ricotta with honey and dash of cinnamon.
- ❖ Then, spread this mixture on the toast.
- ❖ Now, top with fig and sesame seeds.
- ❖ Serve.

9) QUICK SPINACH, FETA WITH EGG BREAKFAST QUESADILLAS

	Cooking Time: 15 Minutes	Servings: 5

- ✓ 8 eggs (optional)
- ✓ 2 tsp olive oil
- ✓ 1 red bell pepper
- ✓ 1/2 red onion
- ✓ 1/4 cup milk
- ✓ 4 handfuls of spinach leaves
- ✓ 1 1/2 cup mozzarella cheese
- ✓ 5 sun-dried tomato tortillas
- ✓ 1/2 cup feta
- ✓ 1/4 tsp salt
- ✓ 1/4 tsp pepper
- ✓ Spray oil

- ❖ In a large non-stick pan over medium heat, add the olive oil
- ❖ Once heated, add the bell pepper and onion, cook for 4-5 minutes until soft
- ❖ In the meantime, whisk together the eggs, milk, salt and pepper in a bowl
- ❖ Add in the egg/milk mixture into the pan with peppers and onions, stirring frequently, until eggs are almost cooked through
- ❖ Add in the spinach and feta, fold into the eggs, stirring until spinach is wilted and eggs are cooked through
- ❖ Remove the eggs from heat and plate
- ❖ Spray a separate large non-stick pan with spray oil, and place over medium heat
- ❖ Add the tortilla, on one half of the tortilla, spread about ½ cup of the egg mixture
- ❖ Top the eggs with around ⅓ cup of shredded mozzarella cheese
- ❖ Fold the second half of the tortilla over, then cook for 2 minutes, or until golden brown
- ❖ Flip and cook for another minute until golden brown
- ❖ Allow the quesadilla to cool completely, divide among the container, store for 2 days or wrap in plastic wrap and foil, and freeze for up to 2 months
- ❖ To Serve: Reheat in oven at 375 for 3-5 minutes or until heated through

10) BREAKFAST COBBLER

	Cooking Time: 12 Minutes	Servings: 4

Ingredients:

- ✓ 2 lbs apples, cut into chunks
- ✓ 1 1/2 cups water
- ✓ 1/4 tsp nutmeg
- ✓ 1 1/2 tsp cinnamon
- ✓ 1/2 cup dry buckwheat
- ✓ 1/2 cup dates, chopped
- ✓ Pinch of ground ginger

Directions:

- ❖ Spray instant pot from inside with cooking spray.
- ❖ Add all ingredients into the instant pot and stir well.
- ❖ Seal pot with a lid and select manual and set timer for 12 minutes.
- ❖ Once done, release pressure using quick release. Remove lid.
- ❖ Stir and serve.

Nutrition: Calories: 195;Fat: 0.9 g;Carbohydrates: 48.3 g;Sugar: 25.8 g;Protein: 3.3 g;Cholesterol: 0 mg

11)

12) EGG QUINOA AND KALE BOWL

	Cooking Time: 5 Minutes	Servings: 2

Ingredients:

- ✓ 1-ounce pancetta, chopped
- ✓ 1 bunch kale, sliced
- ✓ ½ cup cherry tomatoes, halved
- ✓ 1 tsp red wine vinegar
- ✓ 1 cup cooked quinoa
- ✓ 1 tsp olive oil
- ✓ 2 eggs
- ✓ 1/3 cup avocado, sliced
- ✓ sea salt or plain salt
- ✓ fresh black pepper

Directions:

- ❖ Start by heating pancetta in a skillet until golden brown. Add in kale and further cook for 2 minutes.
- ❖ Then, stir in tomatoes, vinegar, and salt and remove from heat.
- ❖ Now, divide this mixture into 2 bowls, add avocado to both, and then set aside.
- ❖ Finally, cook both the eggs and top each bowl with an egg.
- ❖ Serve hot with toppings of your choice.

13) GREEK STRAWBERRY COLD YOGURT

	Cooking Time: 2-4 Hours	Servings: 5

Ingredients:

- ✓ 3 cups plain Greek low-fat yogurt
- ✓ 1 cup sugar
- ✓ ¼ cup lemon juice, freshly squeezed
- ✓ 2 tsp vanilla
- ✓ 1/8 tsp salt
- ✓ 1 cup strawberries, sliced

Directions:

- ❖ In a medium-sized bowl, add yogurt, lemon juice, sugar, vanilla, and salt.
- ❖ Whisk the whole mixture well.
- ❖ Freeze the yogurt mix in a 2-quart ice cream maker according to the given instructions.
- ❖ During the final minute, add the sliced strawberries.
- ❖ Transfer the yogurt to an airtight container.
- ❖ Place in the freezer for 2-4 hours.
- ❖ Remove from the freezer and allow it to stand for 5-15 minutes.
- ❖ Serve and enjoy!

14) SPECIAL PEACH ALMOND OATMEAL

	Cooking Time: 10 Minutes	Servings: 2

- ✓ 1 cup unsweetened almond milk
- ✓ 2 cups of water
- ✓ 1 cup oats
- ✓ 2 peaches, diced
- ✓ Pinch of salt

- ❖ Spray instant pot from inside with cooking spray.
- ❖ Add all ingredients into the instant pot and stir well.
- ❖ Seal pot with a lid and select manual and set timer for 10 minutes.
- ❖ Once done, allow to release pressure naturally for 10 minutes then release remaining using quick release. Remove lid. Stir and serve.

15) EVERYDAY BANANA PEANUT BUTTER PUDDING

	Cooking Time: 25 Minutes	Servings: 1

- ✓ 2 bananas, halved
- ✓ ¼ cup smooth peanut butter
- ✓ Coconut for garnish, shredded

- ❖ Start by blending bananas and peanut butter in a blender and mix until smooth or desired texture obtained.
- ❖ Pour into a bowl and garnish with coconut if desired. Enjoy.

16) SPECIAL COCONUT BANANA MIX

	Cooking Time: 4 Minutes	Servings: 4

✓ 1 cup coconut milk ✓ 1 banana ✓ 1 cup dried coconut ✓ 2 tbsp ground flax seed	✓ 3 tbsp chopped raisins ✓ ⅛ tsp nutmeg ✓ ⅛ tsp cinnamon ✓ Salt to taste	❖ Set a large skillet on the stove and set it to low heat. Chop up the banana. ❖ Pour the coconut milk, nutmeg, and cinnamon into the skillet. ❖ Pour in the ground flaxseed while stirring continuously. ❖ Add the dried coconut and banana. Mix the ingredients until combined well. Allow the mixture to simmer for 2 to 3 minutes while stirring occasionally. Set four airtight containers on the counter. ❖ Remove the pan from heat and sprinkle enough salt for your taste buds. ❖ Divide the mixture into the containers and place them into the fridge overnight. They can remain in the fridge for up to 3 days. ❖ Before you set this tasty mixture in the microwave to heat up, you need to let it thaw on the counter for a bit.

17) RASPBERRY AND LEMON MUFFINS WITH OLIVE OIL

	Cooking Time: 20 Minutes	Servings: 12

✓ Cooking spray to grease baking liners ✓ 1 cup all-purpose flour ✓ 1 cup whole-wheat flour ✓ ½ cup tightly packed light brown sugar ✓ ½ tsp baking soda ✓ ½ tsp aluminum-free baking powder	✓ ⅛ tsp kosher salt ✓ 1¼ cups buttermilk ✓ 1 large egg ✓ ¼ cup extra-virgin olive oil ✓ 1 tbsp freshly squeezed lemon juice ✓ Zest of 2 lemons ✓ 1¼ cups frozen raspberries (do not thaw)	❖ Preheat the oven to 400°F and line a muffin tin with baking liners. Spray the liners lightly with cooking spray. ❖ In a large mixing bowl, whisk together the all-purpose flour, whole-wheat flour, brown sugar, baking soda, baking powder, and salt. ❖ In a medium bowl, whisk together the buttermilk, egg, oil, lemon juice, and lemon zest. ❖ Pour the wet ingredients into the dry ingredients and stir just until blended. Do not overmix. ❖ Fold in the frozen raspberries. ❖ Scoop about ¼ cup of batter into each muffin liner and bake for 20 minutes, or until the tops look browned and a paring knife comes out clean when inserted. Remove the muffins from the tin to cool. ❖ STORAGE: Store covered containers at room temperature for up to 4 days. To freeze muffins for up to 3 months, wrap them in foil and place in an airtight resealable bag.

18) EASY COUSCOUS PEARL SALAD

	Cooking Time: 10 Minutes	Servings: 6

✓ lemon juice, 1 large lemon ✓ 1/3 cup extra-virgin olive oil ✓ 1 tsp dill weed ✓ 1 tsp garlic powder ✓ salt ✓ pepper ✓ 2 cups Pearl Couscous ✓ 2 tbsp extra virgin olive oil ✓ 2 cups grape tomatoes, halved ✓ water as needed	✓ 1/3 cup red onions, finely chopped ✓ ½ English cucumber, finely chopped ✓ 1 15-ounce can chickpeas ✓ 1 14-ounce can artichoke hearts, roughly chopped ✓ ½ cup pitted Kalamata olives ✓ 15-20 pieces fresh basil leaves, roughly torn and chopped ✓ 3 ounces fresh mozzarella	❖ Start by preparing the vinaigrette by mixing all Ingredients: in a bowl. Set aside. Heat olive oil in a medium-sized heavy pot over medium heat. ❖ Add couscous and cook until golden brown. ❖ Add 3 cups of boiling water and cook the couscous according to package instructions. ❖ Once done, drain in a colander and put it to the side. ❖ In a large mixing bowl, add the rest of the Ingredients: except the cheese and basil. ❖ Add the cooked couscous, basil, and mix everything well. ❖ Give the vinaigrette a gentle stir and whisk it into the couscous salad. Mix well. ❖ Adjust/add seasoning as desired. ❖ Add mozzarella cheese. ❖ Garnish with some basil. Enjoy!

19) EGG CUPS WITH TOMATO AND MUSHROOMS

	Cooking Time: 5 Minutes	Servings: 4

Ingredients		Directions
✓ 4 eggs ✓ 1/2 cup tomatoes, chopped ✓ 1/2 cup mushrooms, chopped ✓ 2 tbsp fresh parsley, chopped	✓ 1/4 cup half and half ✓ 1/2 cup cheddar cheese, shredded ✓ Pepper ✓ Salt	❖ In a bowl, whisk the egg with half and half, pepper, and salt. ❖ Add tomato, mushrooms, parsley, and cheese and stir well. ❖ Pour egg mixture into the four small jars and seal jars with lid. ❖ Pour 1 1/2 cups of water into the instant pot then place steamer rack in the pot. ❖ Place jars on top of the steamer rack. ❖ Seal pot with lid and cook on high for 5 minutes. ❖ Once done, release pressure using quick release. Remove lid. ❖ Serve and enjoy.

20) ITALIAN SALAD FOR BREAKFAST

	Cooking Time: 10 Minutes	Servings: 2

Ingredients		Directions:
✓ 4 eggs (optional) ✓ 10 cups arugula ✓ 1/2 seedless cucumber, chopped ✓ 1 cup cooked quinoa, cooled ✓ 1 large avocado ✓ 1 cup natural almonds, chopped	✓ 1/2 cup mixed herbs like mint and dill, chopped ✓ 2 cups halved cherry tomatoes and/or heirloom tomatoes cut into wedges ✓ Extra virgin olive oil ✓ 1 lemon ✓ Sea salt, to taste ✓ Freshly ground black pepper, to taste	❖ Cook the eggs by soft-boiling them - Bring a pot of water to a boil, then reduce heat to a simmer. Gently lower all the eggs into water and allow them to simmer for 6 minutes. Remove the eggs from water and run cold water on top to stop the cooking, process set aside and peel when ready to use ❖ In a large bowl, combine the arugula, tomatoes, cucumber, and quinoa ❖ Divide the salad among 2 containers, store in the fridge for 2 days ❖ To Serve: Garnish with the sliced avocado and halved egg, sprinkle herbs and almonds over top. Drizzle with olive oil, season with salt and pepper, toss to combine. Season with more salt and pepper to taste, a squeeze of lemon juice, and a drizzle of olive oil

21) SPICED PEACH AND ORANGE COMPOTE WITH WHOLE WHEAT PANCAKES

	Cooking Time: 15 Minutes	Servings: 6

Ingredients:		Directions
✓ 1½ cups whole-wheat flour ✓ 1 tsp baking powder ✓ ½ tsp baking soda ✓ ½ tsp ground cinnamon ✓ ⅛ tsp kosher salt ✓ 1 large egg ✓ 1 cup low-fat (2%) plain Greek yogurt	✓ 1 tbsp honey ✓ 1 cup low-fat (2%) milk ✓ 2 tsp olive oil, divided ✓ 1 (10-ounce) package frozen sliced peaches ✓ ½ cup orange juice ✓ ¼ tsp pumpkin pie spice	❖ TO MAKE THE PANCAKES ❖ Combine the flour, baking powder, baking soda, cinnamon, and salt in a large mixing bowl and whisk to make sure everything is distributed evenly. In a separate bowl, whisk together the egg, yogurt, honey, and milk. Pour the liquid ingredients into the dry ingredients and stir until just combined. Do not overmix. ❖ Heat ½ tsp of oil in a 12-inch skillet or griddle over medium heat. Once the pan is hot, spoon ¼ cup of pancake batter into the pan. You should be able to fit pancakes in a 12-inch skillet. Cook each side for about 1 minute and 30 seconds, watching carefully and checking the underside for a golden but not burnt color before flipping. Repeat until all the batter has been used. Place 2 pancakes in each of 6 containers. ❖ TO MAKE THE COMPOTE ❖ Thaw the peaches in the microwave just to the point that they can be cut, about 30 seconds on high. Cut the peaches into 1-inch pieces. ❖ Bring the peaches, orange juice, and pumpkin pie spice to a boil in a saucepan. As soon as bubbles appear, lower the heat to medium-low and cook for 12 minutes, until the juice has thickened and the peaches are very soft. Allow to cool, then mash with a potato masher. ❖ Place 2 tbsp of compote in each of 6 sauce containers.

22) GREEK YOGURT WITH PEANUT BUTTER AND BANANA

	Cooking Time: 5 Minutes	Servings: 4

Ingredients		Directions
✓ 3 cups vanilla Greek yogurt ✓ 2 medium bananas sliced	✓ 1/4 cup creamy natural peanut butter ✓ 1/4 cup flaxseed meal ✓ 1 tsp nutmeg	❖ Divide yogurt between four jars with lids ❖ Top with banana slices ❖ In a bowl, melt the peanut butter in a microwave safe bowl for -40 seconds and drizzle one tbsp on each bowl on top of the bananas ❖ Store in the fridge for up to 3 days ❖ When ready to serve, sprinkle with flaxseed meal and ground nutmeg ❖ Enjoy!

23) SHAKSHUKA WITH VEGETABLES

	Cooking Time: 15 Minutes	Servings: 2

Ingredients		Directions
✓ 1 tbsp olive oil ✓ 1 onion, peeled and diced ✓ 1 clove garlic, peeled and finely minced ✓ 3 cups broccoli rabe, chopped ✓ 3 cups baby spinach leaves ✓ 2 tbsp whole milk or cream	✓ 1 tsp ground cumin ✓ 1/4 tsp black pepper ✓ 1/4 tsp salt (or to taste) ✓ 4 Eggs ✓ Garnish: ✓ 1 pinch sea salt ✓ 1 pinch red pepper flakes	❖ Pre-heat the oven to 350 degrees F ❖ Add the broccoli rabe to a large pot of boiling water, cook for minutes, drain and set aside ❖ In a large oven-proof skillet or cast-iron pan over medium heat, add in the tbsp of olive oil along with the diced onions, cook for about 10 minutes or until the onions become translucent ❖ Add the minced garlic and continue cooking for about another minute ❖ Cut the par-cooked broccoli rabe into small pieces, stir into the onion and garlic mixture ❖ Cook for a couple of minutes, then stir in the baby spinach leaves, continue to cook for a couple more minutes, stirring often, until the spinach begins to wilt ❖ Stir in the ground cumin, salt, ground black pepper, and milk ❖ Make four wells in the mixture, crack an egg into each well – be careful not to break the yolks. Also, note that it's easier to crack each egg into a small bowl and then transfer them to the pan ❖ Place the pan with the eggs into the pre-heated oven, cook for 10 to 15 minutes until the eggs are set to preference ❖ Sprinkle the cooked eggs with a dash of sea salt and a pinch of red pepper flakes ❖ Allow to cool, distribute among the containers, store for 2-3 days ❖ To Serve: Microwave for 1-minute 0r until heated through, serve with crusty whole-wheat bread or warmed slices of pita or naan

24) TASTY COOKIES FOR BREAKFAST

	Cooking Time: 20 Minutes	Servings: 4

Ingredients		Directions
✓ 2 cups oats (rolled) ✓ 1 cup whole wheat flour ✓ 1/4 cup flax seed ✓ 2½ tsp cinnamon (ground) ✓ 1 cup honey	✓ ½ tsp baking soda ✓ 2 egg whites ✓ ½ tsp vanilla extract ✓ 4 tbsp almond butter ✓ pinch of salt	❖ Preheat oven to 325 degrees F. ❖ Whisk oats, flour, flaxseed, cinnamon, salt, and baking soda together in a bowl. ❖ Then, stir honey, egg whites, almond butter, and vanilla extract into the oats mixture until dough is blended. ❖ Now, prepare the baking sheets and scoop the dough in them. ❖ Finally, bake for about 20 minutes. ❖ Serve warm or room temperature.

25) OMELETTE WITH BROCCOLI AND CHEESE

	Cooking Time: 30 Minutes	Servings: 4

Ingredients	Ingredients	Directions
✓ 6 eggs ✓ 2 ½ cups of broccoli florets ✓ ¼ cup of milk ✓ 1 tbsp olive oil ✓ ⅓ cup Romano cheese, grated	✓ ¼ tsp pepper ✓ ⅕ tsp salt ✓ ⅓ cup Greek olives, sliced ✓ Parsley and more Romano cheese for garnish	❖ Turn your oven to broil. ❖ Set a steamer basket in a large pan and add 1 inch of water. ❖ Add the broccoli to the steamer basket and turn the range to medium. Once the water starts to boil, reduce the temperature to low. Steam the broccoli for 4 to 5 minutes. You will know the vegetable is done when it is soft and tender. ❖ In a large bowl, whisk the eggs. ❖ Pour in the milk, pepper, and salt. ❖ Once the broccoli is done, toss into the large bowl and add the olives and grated cheese. ❖ Grease an oven-proof 10-inch skillet and turn the heat on the burner to medium. ❖ Add in the egg mixture, then cook for 4 to 5 minutes. ❖ Set the skillet into the oven but make sure it's at least 4 inches from the heating source. Broil the eggs for 3 minutes. If the eggs are not completely set, continue cooking for another minute or two. ❖ Remove the eggs from the oven and set on the stove so they can cool for a few minutes. ❖ Garnish the Omelette with cheese and parsley. Then, cut into wedges and enjoy!

Nutrition: calories: 229, fats: 17 grams, carbohydrates: 5 grams, protein: 15 grams.

26) BOWL OF GREEK YOGURT FOR BREAKFAST

	Cooking Time: 5 Minutes	Servings: 1

Ingredients	Ingredients	Directions
✓ 1 cup Greek Yogurt plain	✓ 13 cup Pomegranate Seeds (or fresh fruit of your choice) ✓ 1 tsp honey	❖ In a jar with a lid, add the Greek yogurt in a bowl top with fruit and drizzle honey over the top ❖ Close the lid and refrigerate for 3 days

Nutrition: Calories116;Carbs 24g;Total Fat 1.2g;Protein 4g

27) CUCUMBER, CELERY AND LIME SMOOTHIE

	Cooking Time: 15 Minutes	Servings: 2

Ingredients	Ingredients	Directions
✓ 8 stalks of celery, chopped ✓ 1 lemon, juiced	✓ 2 cucumbers, peeled and chopped ✓ ½ cup ice ✓ sweetener of your choice ✓ 1 cup water	❖ Place all the Ingredients: in a blender. ❖ Blend well until smooth and frothy or desired texture. ❖ Serve chilled. ❖ Enjoy.

Nutrition: Calories: 64, Total Fat: 0., Saturated Fat: 0.2, Cholesterol: 0 mg, Sodium: 63 mg, Total Carbohydrate: 15.7 g, Dietary Fiber: 3.4 g, Total Sugars: 6.7 g,

Protein: 2.8 g, Vitamin D: 0 mcg, Calcium: 85 mg, Iron: 1 mg, Potassium: 660 mg

28) BANANA BREAD WITH ALMONDS AND CHOCOLATE

	Cooking Time: 25 Minutes	Servings: 4

Ingredients:

- ✓ Cooking spray or oil to grease the pan
- ✓ 1 cup almond meal
- ✓ 2 large eggs
- ✓ 2 very ripe bananas, mashed
- ✓ 1 tbsp plus 2 tsp maple syrup
- ✓ ½ tsp vanilla extract
- ✓ ½ tsp baking powder
- ✓ ¼ tsp ground cardamom
- ✓ ⅓ cup dark chocolate chips, very roughly chopped

Directions:

- ❖ Preheat the oven to 350°F and spray an 8-inch cake pan or baking dish with cooking spray or rub with oil.
- ❖ Combine all the ingredients in a large mixing bowl. Then pour the mixture into the prepared pan.
- ❖ Place the pan in the oven and bake for 25 minutes. The edges should be browned, and a paring knife should come out clean when the banana bread is pierced.
- ❖ When cool, slice into wedges and place 1 wedge in each of 4 containers.
- ❖ STORAGE: Store covered containers at room temperature for up to 2 days, refrigerate for up to 7 days, or freeze for up to 3 months.

Nutrition: Total calories: 3; Total fat: 23g; Saturated fat: 6g; Sodium: 105mg; Carbohydrates: 37g; Fiber: 6g; Protein: 10g

29) EGG WHITE SANDWICH WITH ITALIAN BREAKFAST

	Cooking Time: 30 Minutes	Servings: 1

- ✓ 1 tsp vegan butter
- ✓ ¼ cup egg whites
- ✓ 1 tsp chopped fresh herbs such as parsley, basil, rosemary
- ✓ 1 whole grain seeded ciabatta roll
- ✓ 1 tbsp pesto
- ✓ 1-2 slices muenster cheese (or other cheese such as provolone, Monterey Jack, etc.)
- ✓ About ½ cup roasted tomatoes
- ✓ Salt, to taste
- ✓ Pepper, to taste
- ✓ Roasted Tomatoes:
- ✓ 10 oz grape tomatoes
- ✓ 1 tbsp extra virgin olive oil
- ✓ Kosher salt, to taste
- ✓ Coarse black pepper, to taste

- ❖ In a small nonstick skillet over medium heat, melt the vegan butter
- ❖ Pour in egg whites, season with salt and pepper, sprinkle with fresh herbs, cook for 3-4 minutes or until egg is done, flip once
- ❖ In the meantime, toast the ciabatta bread in toaster
- ❖ Once done, spread both halves with pesto
- ❖ Place the egg on the bottom half of sandwich roll, folding if necessary, top with cheese, add the roasted tomatoes and top half of roll sandwich
- ❖ To make the roasted tomatoes: Preheat oven to 400 degrees F. Slice tomatoes in half lengthwise. Then place them onto a baking sheet and drizzle with the olive oil, toss to coat. Season with salt and pepper and roast in oven for about 20 minutes, until the skin appears wrinkled

Nutrition: Calories:458;Total Carbohydrates: 51g;Total Fat: 0g;Protein: 21g

30) APRICOT AND STRAWBERRY SMOOTHIE

	Cooking Time: 15 Minutes	Servings: 2

- ✓ 1 cup strawberries, frozen
- ✓ ¾ cup almond milk, unsweetened
- ✓ 2 apricots, pitted and sliced

- ❖ Put all the Ingredients: into the blender.
- ❖ Blend them for a minute or until you reach desired foamy texture.
- ❖ Serve the smoothie.
- ❖ Enjoy.

31) ITALIAN -STYLE VEGGIE QUICHE		
	Cooking Time: 55 Minutes	**Servings:** 8

Ingredients:

- ✓ 1/2 cup sundried tomatoes - dry or in olive oil*
- ✓ Boiling water
- ✓ 1 prepared pie crust
- ✓ 2 tbsp vegan butter
- ✓ 1 onion, diced
- ✓ 2 cloves garlic, minced
- ✓ 1 red pepper, diced
- ✓ 1/4 cup sliced Kalamata olives
- ✓ 1 tsp dried oregano
- ✓ 1 tsp dried parsley
- ✓ 1/3 cup crumbled feta cheese
- ✓ 4 large eggs
- ✓ 1 1/4 cup milk
- ✓ 2 cups fresh spinach or 1/2 cup frozen spinach, thawed and squeezed dry
- ✓ Salt, to taste
- ✓ Pepper, to taste
- ✓ 1 cup shredded cheddar cheese, divided

Directions:

- ❖ If you're using dry sundried tomatoes - In a measure cup, add the sundried tomatoes and pour the boiling water over until just covered, allow to sit for 5 minutes or until the tomatoes are soft. The drain and chop tomatoes, set aside
- ❖ Preheat oven to 375 degrees F
- ❖ Fit a 9-inch pie plate with the prepared pie crust, then flute edges, and set aside
- ❖ In a skillet over medium high heat, melt the butter
- ❖ Add in the onion and garlic, and cook until fragrant and tender, about 3 minutes
- ❖ Add in the red pepper, cook for an additional 3 minutes, or until the peppers are just tender
- ❖ Add in the spinach, olives, oregano, and parsley, cook until the spinach is wilted (if you're using fresh) or heated through (if you're using frozen), about 5 minutes
- ❖ Remove the pan from heat, stir in the feta cheese and tomatoes, spoon the mixture into the prepared pie crust, spreading out evenly, set aside
- ❖ In a medium-sized mixing bowl, whisk together the eggs, 1/2 cup of the cheddar cheese, milk, salt, and pepper
- ❖ Pour this egg and cheese mixture evenly over the spinach mixture in the pie crust
- ❖ Sprinkle top with the remaining cheddar cheese
- ❖ Bake for 50-55 minutes, or until the crust is golden brown and the egg is set
- ❖ Allow to cool completely before slicing
- ❖ Wrap the slices in plastic wrap and then aluminum foil and place in the freezer.
- ❖ To Serve: Remove the aluminum foil and plastic wrap, and microwave for 2 minutes, then allow to rest for 30 seconds, enjoy!
- ❖ Recipe Notes: You'll find two types of sundried tomatoes available in your local grocery store—dry ones and ones packed in olive oil. Both will work for this recipe.
- ❖ If you decide to use dry ones, follow the directions in the recipe to reconstitute them. If you're using oil-packed sundried tomatoes, skip the first step and just remove them from the oil, chop them, and continue with the recipe.
- ❖ Season carefully! Between the feta, cheddar, and olives, this recipe is naturally salty.

Nutrition: Calories:239;Carbs: ;Total Fat: 15g;Protein: 7g

32) SCRAMBLED EGGS ITALIAN STYLE

	Cooking Time: 10 Minutes	Servings: 2

Ingredients:

- ✓ 1 tbsp oil
- ✓ 1 yellow pepper, diced
- ✓ 2 spring onions, sliced
- ✓ 8 cherry tomatoes, quartered
- ✓ 2 tbsp sliced black olives
- ✓ 1 tbsp capers
- ✓ 4 eggs
- ✓ 1/4 tsp dried oregano
- ✓ Black pepper
- ✓ Topping:
- ✓ Fresh parsley, to serve

Directions:

- ❖ In a frying pan over medium heat, add the oil
- ❖ Once heated, add the diced pepper and chopped spring onions, cook for a few minutes, until slightly soft
- ❖ Add in the quartered tomatoes, olives and capers, and cook for 1 more minute
- ❖ Crack the eggs into the pan, immediately scramble with a spoon or spatula
- ❖ Sprinkle with oregano and plenty of black pepper, and stir until the eggs are fully cooked
- ❖ Distribute the eggs evenly into the containers, store in the fridge for 2-3 days
- ❖ To Serve: Reheat in the microwave for 30 seconds or in a toaster oven until warmed through

Nutrition: Calories:249;Carbs: 13g;Total Fat: 17g;Protein: 14g

33) PUDDING WITH CHIA

	Cooking Time: 15 Minutes	Servings: 2

Ingredients:

- ✓ ½ cup chia seeds
- ✓ 2 cups milk
- ✓ 1 tbsp honey

Directions:

- ❖ Combine and mix the chia seeds, milk, and honey in a bowl.
- ❖ Put the mixture in the freezer and let it set.
- ❖ Take the pudding out of the freezer only when you see that the pudding has thickened.
- ❖ Serve chilled.

Nutrition: Calories: 429, Total Fat: 22.4g, Saturated Fat: 4.9, Cholesterol: 20 mg, Sodium: 124 mg, Total Carbohydrate: 44.g, Dietary Fiber: 19.5 g, Total Sugars:

19.6 g, Protein: 17.4 g, Vitamin D: 1 mcg, Calcium: 648 mg, Iron: 4 mg, Potassium: 376 mg

34) RICE BOWLS FOR BREAKFAST

	Cooking Time: 8 Minutes	Servings: 4

Ingredients:

- ✓ 1 cup of brown rice
- ✓ 1 tsp ground cinnamon
- ✓ 1/4 cup almonds, sliced
- ✓ 2 tbsp sunflower seeds
- ✓ 1/4 cup pecans, chopped
- ✓ 1/4 cup walnuts, chopped
- ✓ 2 cup unsweetened almond milk
- ✓ Pinch of salt

Directions:

- ❖ Spray instant pot from inside with cooking spray.
- ❖ Add all ingredients into the instant pot and stir well.
- ❖ Seal pot with lid and cook on high for 8 minutes.
- ❖ Once done, allow to release pressure naturally for 5 minutes then release remaining using quick release. Remove lid.
- ❖ Stir well and serve.

Nutrition: Calories: 291;Fat: 12 g;Carbohydrates: 40.1 g;Sugar: 0.4 g;Protein: 7.g;Cholesterol: 0 mg

35) GREEK YOGURT AND BLUEBERRY PANCAKE

	Cooking Time: 15 Minutes	**Servings:** 6

- ✓ 1 1/4 cup all-purpose flour
- ✓ 2 tsp baking powder
- ✓ 1 tsp baking soda
- ✓ 1/4 tsp salt
- ✓ 1/4 cup sugar
- ✓ 3 eggs
- ✓ 3 tbsp vegan butter unsalted, melted
- ✓ 1/2 cup milk
- ✓ 1 1/2 cups Greek yogurt plain, non-fat
- ✓ 1/2 cup blueberries optional
- ✓ Toppings:
- ✓ Greek yogurt
- ✓ Mixed berries – blueberries, raspberries and blackberries

- ❖ In a large bowl, whisk together the flour, salt, baking powder and baking soda
- ❖ In a separate bowl, whisk together butter, sugar, eggs, Greek yogurt, and milk until the mixture is smooth
- ❖ Then add in the Greek yogurt mixture from step to the dry mixture in step 1, mix to combine, allow the patter to sit for 20 minutes to get a smooth texture – if using blueberries fold them into the pancake batter
- ❖ Heat the pancake griddle, spray with non-stick butter spray or just brush with butter
- ❖ Pour the batter, in 1/4 cupful's, onto the griddle
- ❖ Cook until the bubbles on top burst and create small holes, lift up the corners of the pancake to see if they're golden browned on the bottom
- ❖ With a wide spatula, flip the pancake and cook on the other side until lightly browned
- ❖ Distribute the pancakes in among the storage containers, store in the fridge for 3 day or in the freezer for 2 months
- ❖ To Serve: Reheat microwave for 1 minute (until 80% heated through) or on the stove top, drizzle warm syrup on top, scoop of Greek yogurt, and mixed berries (including blueberries, raspberries, blackberries)

Nutrition: Calories:258;Total Carbohydrates: 33g;Total Fat: 8g;Protein: 11g

36) VEGETABLE BOWL FOR BREAKFAST

	Cooking Time: 5 Minutes	**Servings:** 2

- ✓ Breakfast Bowl:
- ✓ 1 ½ cups cooked quinoa
- ✓ 1 lb asparagus[1], cut into bite-sized pieces, ends trimmed and discarded
- ✓ 1 tbsp avocado oil or olive oil
- ✓ 3 cups shredded kale leaves
- ✓ 1 batch lemony dressing
- ✓ 3 cups shredded, uncooked Brussels sprouts
- ✓ 1 avocado, peeled, pitted and thinly-sliced
- ✓ 4 eggs, cooked to your preference (optional)
- ✓ Garnishes:
- ✓ Toasted sesame seeds
- ✓ Crushed red pepper
- ✓ Sunflower seeds
- ✓ Sliced almonds
- ✓ Hummus
- ✓ Lemon Dressing:
- ✓ 2 tsp Dijon mustard
- ✓ 1 garlic clove, minced
- ✓ 2 tbsp avocado oil or olive oil
- ✓ 2 tbsp freshly-squeezed lemon juice
- ✓ Salt, to taste
- ✓ Freshly-cracked black pepper, to taste

- ❖ In a large sauté pan over medium-high heat, add the oil
- ❖ Once heated, add the asparagus and sauté for 4-5 minutes, stirring occasionally, until tender. Remove from heat and set side
- ❖ Add the Brussels sprouts, quinoa, and cooked asparagus, and toss until combined
- ❖ Distribute among the container, store in fridge for 2-3 days
- ❖ To serve: In a large, mixing bowl combine the kale and lemony dressing. Use your fingers to massage the dressing into the kale for 2-3 minutes, or until the leaves are dark and softened, set aside. In a small mixing bowl, combine the avocado, lemon juice, dijon mustard, garlic clove, salt, and pepper. Assemble the bowls by smearing a spoonful of hummus along the side of each bowl, then portion the kale salad evenly between the four bowls. Top with the avocado slices, egg, and your desired garnishes
- ❖ Recipe Note: Feel free to sub the asparagus with your favorite vegetable(s), sautéing or roasting them until cooked

Nutrition: Calories:632;Carbs: 52g;Total Fat: 39g;Protein: 24g

37) EGG AND ARTICHOKE CASSEROLE FOR BREAKFAST

Cooking Time: 30 To 35 Minutes	Servings: 8

Ingredients	Ingredients	Instructions
✓ 14 ounces artichoke hearts, if using canned remember to drain them ✓ 16 eggs ✓ 1 cup shredded cheddar cheese ✓ 10 ounces chopped spinach, if frozen make sure it is thawed and well-drained ✓ 1 clove of minced garlic ✓ ½ cup ricotta cheese	✓ ½ cup parmesan cheese ✓ ½ tsp crushed red pepper ✓ 1 tsp sea salt ✓ ½ tsp dried thyme ✓ ¼ cup onion, shaved ✓ ¼ cup milk	❖ Grease a 9 x -inch baking pan or place a piece of parchment paper inside of it. ❖ Turn the temperature on your oven to 350 degrees Fahrenheit. ❖ Crack the eggs into a bowl and whisk them well. ❖ Pour in the milk and whisk the two ingredients together. ❖ Squeeze any excess moisture from the spinach with a paper towel. ❖ Toss the spinach and leafless artichoke hearts into the bowl. Stir until well combined. ❖ Add the cheddar cheese, minced garlic, parmesan cheese, red pepper, sea salt, thyme, and onion into the bowl. Mix until all the ingredients are fully incorporated. ❖ Pour the eggs into the baking pan. ❖ Add the ricotta cheese in even dollops before placing the casserole in the oven. ❖ Set your timer for 30 minutes, but watch the casserole carefully after about 20 minutes. Once the eggs stop jiggling and are cooked, remove the meal from the oven. Let the casserole cool down a bit and enjoy!

Nutrition: calories: 302, fats: 18 grams, carbohydrates: grams, protein: 22 grams.

38) BREAKFAST WITH CAULIFLOWER RICE BOWL

Cooking Time: 12 Minutes	Servings: 6

Ingredients	Ingredients	Instructions
✓ 1 cup cauliflower rice ✓ 1/2 tsp red pepper flakes ✓ 1 1/2 tsp curry powder ✓ 1/2 tbsp ginger, grated	✓ 1 cup vegetable stock ✓ 4 tomatoes, chopped ✓ 3 cups broccoli, chopped ✓ Pepper ✓ Salt	❖ Spray instant pot from inside with cooking spray. ❖ Add all ingredients into the instant pot and stir well. ❖ Seal pot with lid and cook on high for 12 minutes. ❖ Once done, allow to release pressure naturally for 10 minutes then release remaining using quick release. Remove lid. ❖ Stir and serve.

Nutrition: Calories: 44;Fat: 0.8 g;Carbohydrates: 8.2 g;Sugar: 3.8 g;Protein: 2.8 g;Cholesterol: 0 mg

39) SALTED YOGURT WITH CUCUMBER AND DILL

Cooking Time: 10 Minutes	Servings: 4

Ingredients	Ingredients	Instructions
✓ 2 cups low-fat (2%) plain Greek yogurt ✓ 4 tsp minced shallot ✓ 4 tsp freshly squeezed lemon juice ✓ ¼ cup chopped fresh dill	✓ 2 tsp olive oil ✓ ¼ tsp kosher salt ✓ Pinch freshly ground black pepper ✓ 2 cups chopped Persian cucumbers (about 4 medium cucumbers)	❖ Combine the yogurt, shallot, lemon juice, dill, oil, salt, and pepper in a large bowl. Taste the mixture and add another pinch of salt if needed. ❖ Scoop ½ cup of yogurt into each of 4 containers. Place ½ cup of chopped cucumbers in each of 4 separate small containers or resealable sandwich bags. ❖ STORAGE: Store covered containers in the refrigerator for up to 5 days.

Nutrition: Total calories: 127; Total fat: 5g; Saturated fat: 2g; Sodium: 200mg; Carbohydrates: 9g; Fiber: 2g; Protein: 11g

40) GREEK STRAWBERRY COLD YOGURT

	Cooking Time: 2-4 Hours	Servings: 5

Ingredients:

- ✓ 3 cups plain Greek low-fat yogurt
- ✓ 1 cup sugar
- ✓ ¼ cup lemon juice, freshly squeezed
- ✓ 2 tsp vanilla
- ✓ 1/8 tsp salt
- ✓ 1 cup strawberries, sliced

Directions:

- ❖ In a medium-sized bowl, add yogurt, lemon juice, sugar, vanilla, and salt.
- ❖ Whisk the whole mixture well.
- ❖ Freeze the yogurt mix in a 2-quart ice cream maker according to the given instructions.
- ❖ During the final minute, add the sliced strawberries.
- ❖ Transfer the yogurt to an airtight container.
- ❖ Place in the freezer for 2-4 hours.
- ❖ Remove from the freezer and allow it to stand for 5-15 minutes.
- ❖ Serve and enjoy!

Nutrition: Calories: 251, Total Fat: 0.5 g, Saturated Fat: 0.1 g, Cholesterol: 3 mg, Sodium: 130 mg, Total Carbohydrate: 48.7 g, Dietary Fiber: 0.6 g, Total Sugars: 47.3 g, Protein: 14.7 g, Vitamin D: 1 mcg, Calcium: 426 mg, Iron: 0 mg, Potassium: 62 mg

41) SPECIAL PEACH ALMOND OATMEAL

	Cooking Time: 10 Minutes	Servings: 2

Ingredients:

- ✓ 1 cup unsweetened almond milk
- ✓ 2 cups of water
- ✓ 1 cup oats
- ✓ 2 peaches, diced
- ✓ Pinch of salt

Directions:

- ❖ Spray instant pot from inside with cooking spray.
- ❖ Add all ingredients into the instant pot and stir well.
- ❖ Seal pot with a lid and select manual and set timer for 10 minutes.
- ❖ Once done, allow to release pressure naturally for 10 minutes then release remaining using quick release. Remove lid.
- ❖ Stir and serve.

Nutrition: Calories: 234;Fat: 4.8 g;Carbohydrates: 42.7 g;Sugar: 9 g;Protein: 7.3 g;Cholesterol: 0 mg

42) EVERYDAY BANANA PEANUT BUTTER PUDDING

	Cooking Time: 25 Minutes	Servings: 1

Ingredients:

- ✓ 2 bananas, halved
- ✓ ¼ cup smooth peanut butter
- ✓ Coconut for garnish, shredded

Directions:

- ❖ Start by blending bananas and peanut butter in a blender and mix until smooth or desired texture obtained.
- ❖ Pour into a bowl and garnish with coconut if desired.
- ❖ Enjoy.

Nutrition: Calories: 589, Total Fat: 33.3g, Saturated Fat: 6.9, Cholesterol: 0 mg, Sodium: 13 mg, Total Carbohydrate: 66.5 g, Dietary Fiber: 10 g, Total Sugars: 38 g, Protein: 18.8 g, Vitamin D: 0 mcg, Calcium: 40 mg, Iron: 2 mg, Potassium: 1264 mg

Chapter 2. <u>LUNCH</u>

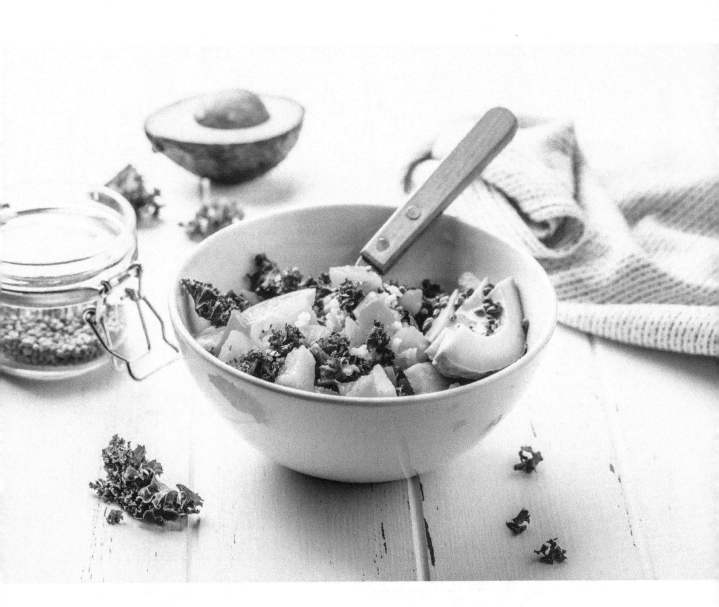

43) SPECIAL FRUIT SALAD WITH MINT AND ORANGE BLOSSOM WATER

	Cooking Time: 10 Minutes	**Servings: 5**

Ingredients:

- ✓ 3 cups cantaloupe, cut into 1-inch cubes
- ✓ 2 cups hulled and halved strawberries
- ✓ ½ tsp orange blossom water
- ✓ 2 tbsp chopped fresh mint

Directions:

- ❖ In a large bowl, toss all the ingredients together.
- ❖ Place 1 cup of fruit salad in each of 5 containers.
- ❖ STORAGE: Store covered containers in the refrigerator for up to 5 days.

Nutrition: Total calories: 52; Total fat: 1g; Saturated fat: <1g; Sodium: 10mg; Carbohydrates: 12g; Fiber: 2g; Protein: 1g

44) ROASTED BROCCOLI WITH RED ONIONS AND POMEGRANATE SEEDS

	Cooking Time: 20 Minutes	**Servings: 5**

Ingredients:

- ✓ 1 (12-ounce) package broccoli florets (about 6 cups)
- ✓ 1 small red onion, thinly sliced
- ✓ 2 tbsp olive oil
- ✓ ¼ tsp kosher salt
- ✓ 1 (5.3-ounce) container pomegranate seeds (1 cup)

Directions:

- ❖ Preheat the oven to 425°F and line 2 sheet pans with silicone baking mats or parchment paper.
- ❖ Place the broccoli and onion on the sheet pans and toss with the oil and salt. Place the pans in the oven and roast for minutes.
- ❖ After removing the pans from the oven, cool the veggies, then toss with the pomegranate seeds.
- ❖ Place 1 cup of veggies in each of 5 containers.
- ❖ STORAGE: Store covered containers in the refrigerator for up to days.

Nutrition: Total calories: 118; Total fat: ; Saturated fat: 1g; Sodium: 142mg; Carbohydrates: 12g; Fiber: 4g; Protein: 2g

45) DELICIOUS CHERMOULA SAUCE

	Cooking Time: 10 Minutes	**Servings: 1 Cup**

Ingredients:

- ✓ 1 cup packed parsley leaves
- ✓ 1 cup cilantro leaves
- ✓ ½ cup mint leaves
- ✓ 1 tsp chopped garlic
- ✓ ½ tsp ground cumin
- ✓ ½ tsp ground coriander
- ✓ ½ tsp smoked paprika
- ✓ ⅛ tsp cayenne pepper
- ✓ ⅛ tsp kosher salt
- ✓ 3 tbsp freshly squeezed lemon juice
- ✓ 3 tbsp water
- ✓ ½ cup extra-virgin olive oil

Directions:

- ❖ Place all the ingredients in a blender or food processor and blend until smooth.
- ❖ Pour the chermoula into a container and refrigerate.
- ❖ STORAGE: Store the covered container in the refrigerator for up to 5 days.

Nutrition: (¼ cup): Total calories: 257; Total fat: 27g; Saturated fat: ; Sodium: 96mg; Carbohydrates: 4g; Fiber: 2g; Protein: 1g

46) DEVILED EGG PESTO WITH SUN-DRIED TOMATOES

	Cooking Time: 15 Minutes	Servings: 5

Ingredients:

- ✓ 5 large eggs
- ✓ 3 tbsp prepared pesto
- ✓ ¼ tsp white vinegar
- ✓ 2 tbsp low-fat (2%) plain Greek yogurt
- ✓ 5 tsp sliced sun-dried tomatoes

❖ Place the eggs in a saucepan and cover with water. Bring the water to a boil. As soon as the water starts to boil, place a lid on the pan and turn the heat off. Set a timer for minutes.

❖ When the timer goes off, drain the hot water and run cold water over the eggs to cool.

❖ Peel the eggs, slice in half vertically, and scoop out the yolks. Place the yolks in a medium mixing bowl and add the pesto, vinegar, and yogurt. Mix well, until creamy.

❖ Scoop about 1 tbsp of the pesto-yolk mixture into each egg half. Top each with ½ tsp of sun-dried tomatoes.

❖ Place 2 stuffed egg halves in each of separate containers.

❖ STORAGE: Store covered containers in the refrigerator for up to 5 days.

47) WHITE BEAN WITH MUSHROOM DIP

	Cooking Time: 8 Minutes	Servings: 3 Cups

Ingredients:

- ✓ 2 tsp olive oil, plus 2 tbsp
- ✓ 8 ounces button or cremini mushrooms, sliced
- ✓ 1 tsp chopped garlic
- ✓ 1 tbsp fresh thyme leaves
- ✓ 2 (15.5-ounce) cans cannellini beans, drained and rinsed
- ✓ 2 tbsp plus 1 tsp freshly squeezed lemon juice
- ✓ ½ tsp kosher salt

❖ Heat 2 tsp of oil in a -inch skillet over medium-high heat. Once the oil is shimmering, add the mushrooms and sauté for 6 minutes. Add the garlic and thyme and continue cooking for 2 minutes.

❖ While the mushrooms are cooking, place the beans and lemon juice, the remaining tbsp of oil, and the salt in the bowl of a food processor. Add the mushrooms as soon as they are done cooking and blend everything until smooth. Scrape down the sides of the bowl if necessary and continue to process until smooth.

❖ Taste and adjust the seasoning with lemon juice or salt if needed.

❖ Scoop the dip into a container and refrigerate.

❖ STORAGE: Store the covered container in the refrigerator for up to days. Dip can be frozen for up to 3 months.

48) SPICY SAUTÉED CABBAGE IN NORTH AFRICAN STYLE

	Cooking Time: 10 Minutes	Servings: 4

Ingredients:

- ✓ 2 tsp olive oil
- ✓ 1 small head green cabbage (about 1½ to 2 pounds), cored and thinly sliced
- ✓ 1 tsp ground coriander
- ✓ 1 tsp garlic powder
- ✓ ½ tsp caraway seeds
- ✓ ½ tsp ground cumin
- ✓ ¼ tsp kosher salt
- ✓ Pinch red chili flakes (optional—if you don't like heat, omit it)
- ✓ 1 tsp freshly squeezed lemon juice

Directions:

❖ Heat the oil in a -inch skillet over medium-high heat. Once the oil is hot, add the cabbage and cook down for 3 minutes. Add the coriander, garlic powder, caraway seeds, cumin, salt, and chili flakes (if using) and stir to combine. Continue cooking the cabbage for about 7 more minutes.

❖ Stir in the lemon juice and cool.

❖ Place 1 heaping cup of cabbage in each of 4 containers.

❖ STORAGE: Store covered containers in the refrigerator for up to 5 days.

49) FLAX, BLUEBERRY, AND SUNFLOWER BUTTER BITES

	Cooking Time: 10 Minutes	Servings: 6

- ✓ ¼ cup ground flaxseed
- ✓ ½ cup unsweetened sunflower butter, preferably unsalted
- ✓ ⅓ cup dried blueberries
- ✓ 2 tbsp all-fruit blueberry preserves
- ✓ Zest of 1 lemon
- ✓ 2 tbsp unsalted sunflower seeds
- ✓ ⅓ cup rolled oats

- ❖ Mix all the ingredients in a medium mixing bowl until well combined.
- ❖ Form 1balls, slightly smaller than a golf ball, from the mixture and place on a plate in the freezer for about 20 minutes to firm up.
- ❖ Place 2 bites in each of 6 containers and refrigerate.
- ❖ STORAGE: Store covered containers in the refrigerator for up to 5 days. Bites may also be stored in the freezer for up to 3 months.

50) SPECIAL DIJON RED WINE VINAIGRETTE

	Cooking Time: 5 Minutes	Servings: ½ Cup

- ✓ 2 tsp Dijon mustard
- ✓ 3 tbsp red wine vinegar
- ✓ 1 tbsp water
- ✓ ¼ tsp dried oregano
- ✓ ¼ tsp chopped garlic
- ✓ ⅛ tsp kosher salt
- ✓ ¼ cup olive oil

- ❖ Place the mustard, vinegar, water, oregano, garlic, and salt in a small bowl and whisk to combine.
- ❖ Whisk in the oil, pouring it into the mustard-vinegar mixture in a thin steam.
- ❖ Pour the vinaigrette into a container and refrigerate.
- ❖ STORAGE: Store the covered container in the refrigerator for up to 2 weeks. Allow the vinaigrette to come to room temperature and shake before serving.

51) DELICIOUS CREAMY KETO CUCUMBER SALAD

	Cooking Time: 5 Minutes	Servings: 2

- ✓ 2 tbsp mayonnaise
- ✓ Salt and black pepper, to taste
- ✓ 1 cucumber, sliced and quartered
- ✓ 2 tbsp lemon juice

- ❖ Mix together the mayonnaise, cucumber slices, and lemon juice in a large bowl.
- ❖ Season with salt and black pepper and combine well.
- ❖ Dish out in a glass bowl and serve while it is cold.

Nutrition: Calories: 8Carbs: 9.3g;Fats: 5.2g;Proteins: 1.2g;Sodium: 111mg;Sugar: 3.8g

52) CABBAGE SOUP WITH SAUSAGE AND MUSHROOMS

	Cooking Time: 1 Hour 10 Minutes	Servings: 6

Ingredients:

- ✓ 2 cups fresh kale, cut into bite sized pieces
- ✓ 6.5 ounces mushrooms, sliced
- ✓ 6 cups chicken bone broth
- ✓ 1 pound sausage, cooked and sliced
- ✓ Salt and black pepper, to taste

Directions:

- ❖ Heat chicken broth with two cans of water in a large pot and bring to a boil.
- ❖ Stir in the rest of the ingredients and allow the soup to simmer on low heat for about 1 hour.
- ❖ Dish out and serve hot.

53) CLASSIC MINESTRONE SOUP

Cooking Time: 25 Minutes	**Servings:** 6

- ✓ 2 tbsp olive oil
- ✓ 3 cloves garlic, minced
- ✓ 1 onion, diced
- ✓ 2 carrots, peeled and diced
- ✓ 2 stalks celery, diced
- ✓ 1 1/2 tsp dried basil
- ✓ 1 tsp dried oregano
- ✓ 1/2 tsp fennel seed
- ✓ 6 cups low sodium chicken broth
- ✓ 1 (28-ounce can diced tomatoes

- ✓ 1 (16-ounce can kidney beans, drained and rinsed
- ✓ 1 zucchini, chopped
- ✓ 1 (3-inch Parmesan rind
- ✓ 1 bay leaf
- ✓ 1 bunch kale leaves, chopped
- ✓ 2 tsp red wine vinegar
- ✓ Kosher salt and black pepper, to taste
- ✓ 1/3 cup freshly grated Parmesan
- ✓ 2 tbsp chopped fresh parsley leaves

- ❖ Preheat olive oil in the insert of the Instant Pot on Sauté mode.
- ❖ Add carrots, celery, and onion, sauté for 3 minutes.
- ❖ Stir in fennel seeds, oregano, and basil. Stir cook for 1 minute.
- ❖ Add stock, beans, tomatoes, parmesan, bay leaf, and zucchini.
- ❖ Secure and seal the Instant Pot lid then select Manual mode to cook for minutes at high pressure.
- ❖ Once done, release the pressure completely then remove the lid.
- ❖ Add kale and let it sit for 2 minutes in the hot soup.
- ❖ Stir in red wine, vinegar, pepper, and salt.
- ❖ Garnish with parsley and parmesan.
- ❖ Enjoy.

54) SPECIAL SALAD OF KOMBU SEAWEED

Cooking Time: 40 Minutes	**Servings:** 6

- ✓ 4 garlic cloves, crushed
- ✓ 1 pound fresh kombu seaweed, boiled and cut into strips

- ✓ 2 tbsp apple cider vinegar
- ✓ Salt, to taste
- ✓ 2 tbsp coconut aminos

- ❖ Mix together the kombu, garlic, apple cider vinegar, and coconut aminos in a large bowl.
- ❖ Season with salt and combine well.
- ❖ Dish out in a glass bowl and serve immediately.

55) TURKEY MEATBALL WITH DITALINI SOUP

Cooking Time: 40 Minutes	**Servings:** 4

- ✓ meatballs:
- ✓ 1 pound 93% lean ground turkey
- ✓ 1/3 cup seasoned breadcrumbs
- ✓ 3 tbsp grated Pecorino Romano cheese
- ✓ 1 large egg, beaten
- ✓ 1 clove crushed garlic
- ✓ 1 tbsp fresh minced parsley
- ✓ 1/2 tsp kosher salt
- ✓ Soup:
- ✓ cooking spray
- ✓ 1 tsp olive oil
- ✓ 1/2 cup chopped onion
- ✓ 1/2 cup chopped celery

- ✓ 1/2 cup chopped carrot
- ✓ 3 cloves minced garlic
- ✓ 1 can (28 ounces diced San Marzano tomatoes
- ✓ 4 cups reduced sodium chicken broth
- ✓ 4 torn basil leaves
- ✓ 2 bay leaves
- ✓ 1 cup ditalini pasta
- ✓ 1 cup zucchini, diced small
- ✓ Parmesan rind, optional
- ✓ Grated parmesan cheese, optional for serving

- ❖ Thoroughly combine turkey with egg, garlic, parsley, salt, pecorino and breadcrumbs in a bowl.
- ❖ Make 30 equal sized meatballs out of this mixture.
- ❖ Preheat olive oil in the insert of the Instant Pot on Sauté mode.
- ❖ Sear the meatballs in the heated oil in batches, until brown.
- ❖ Set the meatballs aside in a plate.
- ❖ Add more oil to the insert of the Instant Pot.
- ❖ Stir in carrots, garlic, celery, and onion. Sauté for 4 minutes.
- ❖ Add basil, bay leaves, tomatoes, and Parmesan rind.
- ❖ Return the seared meatballs to the pot along with the broth.
- ❖ Secure and sear the Instant Pot lid and select Manual mode for 15 minutes at high pressure.
- ❖ Once done, release the pressure completely then remove the lid.
- ❖ Add zucchini and pasta, cook it for 4 minutes on Sauté mode.
- ❖ Garnish with cheese and basil.
- ❖ Serve.

56) NICE COLD AVOCADO AND MINT SOUP

	Cooking Time: 5 Minutes	Servings: 2

Ingredients:

- ✓ 1 cup coconut milk, chilled
- ✓ 1 medium ripe avocado
- ✓ 1 tbsp lime juice
- ✓ Salt, to taste
- ✓ 20 fresh mint leaves

Directions:

- ❖ Put all the ingredients into an immersion blender and blend until a thick mixture is formed.
- ❖ Allow to cool in the fridge for about 10 minutes and serve chilled.

57) CLASSIC SPLIT PEA SOUP

	Cooking Time: 30 Minutes	Servings: 6

Ingredients:

- ✓ 3 tbsp butter
- ✓ 1 onion diced
- ✓ 2 ribs celery diced
- ✓ 2 carrots diced
- ✓ 6 oz. diced ham
- ✓ 1 lb. dry split peas sorted and rinsed
- ✓ 6 cups chicken stock
- ✓ 2 bay leaves
- ✓ kosher salt and black pepper

Directions:

- ❖ Set your Instant Pot on Sauté mode and melt butter in it.
- ❖ Stir in celery, onion, carrots, salt, and pepper.
- ❖ Sauté them for 5 minutes then stir in split peas, ham bone, chicken stock, and bay leaves.
- ❖ Seal and lock the Instant Pot lid then select Manual mode for 15 minutes at high pressure.
- ❖ Once done, release the pressure completely then remove the lid.
- ❖ Remove the ham bone and separate meat from the bone.
- ❖ Shred or dice the meat and return it to the soup.
- ❖ Adjust seasoning as needed then serve warm.
- ❖ Enjoy.

58) BAKED FILLET OF SOLE ITALIAN STYLE

	Cooking Time: 15 Minutes	Servings: 6

Ingredients:

- ✓ 1 lime or lemon, juice of
- ✓ 1/2 cup extra virgin olive oil
- ✓ 3 tbsp unsalted melted vegan butter
- ✓ 2 shallots, thinly sliced
- ✓ 3 garlic cloves, thinly-sliced
- ✓ 2 tbsp capers
- ✓ 1.5 lb Sole fillet, about 10–12 thin fillets
- ✓ 4–6 green onions, top trimmed, halved lengthwise
- ✓ 1 lime or lemon, sliced (optional)
- ✓ 3/4 cup roughly chopped fresh dill for garnish
- ✓ 1 tsp seasoned salt, or to your taste
- ✓ 3/4 tsp ground black pepper
- ✓ 1 tsp ground cumin
- ✓ 1 tsp garlic powder

Directions:

- ❖ Preheat over to 375-degree F
- ❖ In a small bowl, whisk together olive oil, lime juice, and melted butter with a sprinkle of seasoned salt, stir in the garlic, shallots, and capers.
- ❖ In a separate small bowl, mix together the pepper, cumin, seasoned salt, and garlic powder, season the fish fillets each on both sides
- ❖ On a large baking pan or dish, arrange the fish fillets and cover with the buttery lime
- ❖ Arrange the green onion halves and lime slices on top
- ❖ Bake in 375 degrees F for 10-15 minutes, do not overcook
- ❖ Remove the fish fillets from the oven
- ❖ Allow the dish to cool completely
- ❖ Distribute among the containers, store for 2-3 days
- ❖ To Serve: Reheat in the microwave for 1-2 minutes or until heated through. Garnish with the chopped fresh dill. Serve with your favorite and a fresh salad
- ❖ Recipe Notes: If you can't get your hands on a sole fillet, cook this recipe with a different white fish. Just remember to change the baking time since it will be different.

Nutrition: Calories:350;Carbs:7 g;Total Fat: 26g;Protein: 23g

59) BAKED CHICKEN BREAST

	Cooking Time: 50 Minutes	Servings: 2

✓ 2 skinless and boneless chicken breasts (about 8 ounces each) ✓ salt ✓ ground black pepper ✓ ¼ cup olive oil	✓ ¼ cup freshly squeezed lemon juice ✓ 1 garlic clove, minced ✓ ½ tsp dried oregano ✓ ¼ tsp dried thyme	❖ Preheat oven to a temperature of 400 degrees F. ❖ Season the chicken breasts carefully with salt and pepper on all sides. ❖ Place the chicken in a bowl. ❖ Take another bowl and add olive oil, lemon juice, oregano, garlic, and thyme. Mix well to make the marinade. ❖ Pour the marinade on top of chicken breasts and allow to marinate for 10 minutes. Set an oven rack about inches above the heat source. ❖ Place the chicken breasts into a baking pan and pour extra marinade on top. Bake for about 35-45 minutes until the center is no longer pink and the juices run clear. Move the baking dish to top rack and broil for about 5 minutes. Cool, spread over containers with some side dish and enjoy!

60) LEMON FISH GRILL

	Cooking Time: 15 Minutes	Servings: 4

✓ ¼ tsp sea salt ✓ 3 to 4 lemons ✓ ¼ tsp ground black pepper	✓ 4 ounces any fish fillets, such as salmon or cod ✓ 1 tbsp olive oil	❖ Ensure that the fish fillets are dry. If you know or feel they are a bit damp, take a paper towel and pat them dry. ❖ Leave the fish fillets on the counter for 10 minutes so they can stand at room temperature. ❖ Turn on your grill to medium-high heat or set the temperature to 400 degrees Fahrenheit. Using nonstick cooking spray, coat the grill so the fish won't stick. Take one lemon and cut it in half. Set one of the halves aside and cut the remaining half into ¼-inch thick slices. ❖ Now, take the other half of the lemon and squeeze at least 1 tbsp of juice out into a small bowl. Add oil into the small bowl and whisk the ingredients together. Brush the fish with the lemon and oil mixture. Make sure you get both sides of the fish. ❖ Arrange the lemon slices on the grill in the shape of the fish, it might take about 3 to 4 slices for one fish. Place the fish on top of the lemon slices and grill the ingredients together. If you don't have a lid for your grill, cover it with a different lid that will fit or use aluminum foil. ❖ When the fish is about half-way done, turn it over so the other side is laying on top of the lemon slices. You will know the fish is done when it starts to look flaky and separates easily, which you can check by gently pressing a fork onto the fish.

61) BAKED BEANS ITALIAN STYLE

	Cooking Time: 15 To 20 Minutes.	Servings: 6

✓ ½ cup chopped onion ✓ ¼ cup red wine vinegar ✓ ¼ tbsp ground cinnamon ✓ 15 ounces or 2 cans of great northern beans, do not drain	✓ 2 tsp extra virgin olive oil ✓ 12 ounces tomato paste, low sodium ✓ ½ cup water	❖ Turn a burner to medium heat and add oil to a saucepan. ❖ Add the onion and cook for 4 to 5 minutes. Stir well. ❖ Combine the vinegar, tomato paste, cinnamon, and water. Mix until all the ingredients are well combined. ❖ Switch the heat to a low setting. ❖ Using a colander, drain one can of beans and pour into the pan. ❖ Open the second can of beans and pour all of it, including the liquid, into the saucepan and stir. ❖ Continue to cook the beans for 10 minutes while stirring frequently. ❖ Serve and enjoy!

Nutrition: calories: 236, fats: 3 grams, carbohydrates: 42 grams, protein: 10 grams

62) POMODORO TILAPIA

	Cooking Time: 15 Minutes	**Servings:** 4

Ingredients:

- ✓ 3 tbsp sun-dried tomatoes packed in oil, drained (juice/oil reserved) and chopped
- ✓ 1 tbsp capers, drained
- ✓ 2 pieces tilapia
- ✓ 1 tbsp oil from sun-dried tomatoes
- ✓ 1 tbsp lemon juice
- ✓ 2 tbsp Kalamata olives, pitted and chopped

Directions:

- ❖ Preheat oven to 375 degrees F.
- ❖ Add sun-dried tomatoes, capers, and olives to a bowl; stir well and set aside.
- ❖ Place the tilapia fillets side by side on a baking sheet.
- ❖ Drizzle with oil and lemon juice.
- ❖ Bake for about 10-1minutes.
- ❖ Check the fish after 10 minutes to see if they are flakey.
- ❖ Once done, top the fish with tomato mixture.

Nutrition: Calories: , Total Fat: 4.4 g, Saturated Fat: 0.8 g, Cholesterol: 28 mg, Sodium: 122 mg, Total Carbohydrate: 0.8 g, Dietary Fiber: 0.3 g, Total Sugars: 0.3 g, Protein: 10.7 g, Vitamin D: 0 mcg, Calcium: 16 mg, Iron: 1 mg, Potassium: 26 mg

63) LENTIL SOUP WITH CHICKEN

	Cooking Time: 45 Minutes	**Servings:** 4

Ingredients:

- ✓ 1 pound dried lentils
- ✓ 12 ounces boneless chicken thigh meat
- ✓ 7 cups water
- ✓ 1 small onion, diced
- ✓ 2 scallions, chopped
- ✓ ¼ cup chopped cilantro
- ✓ 3 cloves garlic
- ✓ 1 medium tomato, diced
- ✓ 1 tsp garlic powder
- ✓ 1 tsp cumin
- ✓ ¼ tsp oregano
- ✓ ½ tsp paprika
- ✓ ½ tsp kosher salt

Directions:

- ❖ Add all of the listed Ingredients: to your Instant Pot.
- ❖ Set your pot to SOUP mode and cook for 30 minutes.
- ❖ Allow the pressure to release naturally.
- ❖ Take the chicken out and shred.
- ❖ Place the chicken back in the pot and stir.
- ❖ Pour to the jars.
- ❖ Enjoy!

64) ASPARAGUS WRAPPED WITH BACON

	Cooking Time: 30 Minutes	**Servings:** 2

Ingredients:

- ✓ 1/3 cup heavy whipping cream
- ✓ 2 bacon slices, precooked
- ✓ 4 small spears asparagus
- ✓ Salt, to taste
- ✓ 1 tbsp butter

Directions:

- ❖ Preheat the oven to 360 degrees F and grease a baking sheet with butter.
- ❖ Meanwhile, mix cream, asparagus and salt in a bowl.
- ❖ Wrap the asparagus in bacon slices and arrange them in the baking dish.
- ❖ Transfer the baking dish in the oven and bake for about 20 minutes.
- ❖ Remove from the oven and serve hot.
- ❖ Place the bacon wrapped asparagus in a dish and set aside to cool for meal prepping. Divide it in 2 containers and cover the lid. Refrigerate for about 2 days and reheat in the microwave before serving.

Nutrition: Calories: 204 ;Carbohydrates: 1.4g;Protein: 5.9g;Fat: 19.3g;Sugar: 0.5g;Sodium: 291mg

65) COOL ITALIAN-STYLE FISH

	Cooking Time: 30 Minutes	Servings: 8

✓ 6 ounces halibut fillets ✓ 1 tbsp Greek seasoning ✓ 1 large tomato, chopped ✓ 1 onion, chopped ✓ 5 ounces kalamata olives, pitted	✓ ¼ cup capers ✓ ¼ cup olive oil ✓ 1 tbsp lemon juice ✓ Salt and pepper as needed	❖ Pre-heat your oven to 350-degree Fahrenheit ❖ Transfer the halibut fillets on a large aluminum foil Season with Greek seasoning ❖ Take a bowl and add tomato, onion, olives, olive oil, capers, pepper, lemon juice and salt ❖ Mix well and spoon the tomato mix over the halibut Seal the edges and fold to make a packet Place the packet on a baking sheet and bake in your oven for 30-40 minutes Serve once the fish flakes off and enjoy! ❖ Meal Prep/Storage Options: Store in airtight containers in your fridge for 1-2 days.

66) FANCY LUNCHEON SALAD

	Cooking Time: 40 Minutes	Servings: 2

✓ 6-ounce cooked salmon, chopped ✓ 1 tbsp fresh dill, chopped ✓ Salt and black pepper, to taste	✓ 4 hard-boiled grass-fed eggs, peeled and cubed ✓ 2 celery stalks, chopped ✓ ½ yellow onion, chopped ✓ ¾ cup avocado mayonnaise	❖ Put all the ingredients in a bowl and mix until well combined. ❖ Cover with a plastic wrap and refrigerate for about 3 hours to serve. ❖ For meal prepping, put the salad in a container and refrigerate for up to days

Nutrition: Calories: 303 ;Carbohydrates: 1.7g;Protein: 10.3g;Fat: 30g ;Sugar: 1g;Sodium: 31g

67) BEEF SAUTEED WITH MOROCCAN SPICES AND BUTTERNUT SQUASH WITH CHICKPEAS

	Cooking Time: 15 Minutes	Servings: 4

✓ 1 tbsp olive oil, plus 2 tsp ✓ 1 pound precut butternut squash cut into ½-inch cubes ✓ 3 ounces scallions, white and green parts chopped (1 cup) ✓ 1 tbsp water ✓ ¼ tsp baking soda ✓ ¾ pound flank steak, sliced across the grain into ⅛-inch thick slices ✓ ½ tsp garlic powder ✓ ¼ tsp ground ginger ✓ ¼ tsp turmeric	✓ ¼ tsp ground cumin ✓ ¼ tsp ground coriander ✓ ⅛ tsp cayenne pepper ✓ ⅛ tsp ground cinnamon ✓ ½ tsp kosher salt, divided ✓ 1 (14-ounce) can chickpeas, drained and rinsed ✓ ½ cup dried apricots, quartered ✓ ½ cup cilantro leaves, chopped ✓ 2 tsp freshly squeezed lemon juice ✓ 8 tsp sliced almonds	❖ Heat tbsp of oil in a 12-inch skillet. Once the oil is hot, add the squash and scallions, and cook until the squash is tender, about 10 to 12 minutes. ❖ Mix the water and baking soda together in a small prep bowl. Place the beef in a medium bowl, pour the baking-soda water over it, and mix to combine. Let it sit for 5 minutes. ❖ In a small bowl, combine the garlic powder, ginger, turmeric, cumin, coriander, cayenne, cinnamon, and ¼ tsp of salt, then add the mixture to the beef. Stir to combine. ❖ When the squash is tender, turn the heat off and add the remaining ¼ tsp of salt and the chickpeas, dried apricots, cilantro, and lemon juice to taste. Stir to combine. Place the contents of the pan in a bowl to cool. ❖ Clean out the skillet and heat the remaining 2 tsp of oil over high heat. When the oil is hot, add the beef and cook until it is no longer pink, about 2 to 3 minutes. ❖ Place 1¼ cups of the squash mixture and one quarter of the beef slices in each of 4 containers. Sprinkle 2 tsp of sliced almonds over each container. ❖ STORAGE: Store covered containers in the refrigerator for up to 5 days.

Nutrition: Total calories: 404; Total fat: 14g; Saturated fat: 1g; Sodium: 355mg; Carbohydrates: 46g; Fiber: 12g; Protein: 27g

68) NORTH AFRICAN–INSPIRED SAUTÉED SHRIMP AND LEEKS WITH PEPPERS

	Cooking Time: 20 Minutes	Servings: 4

Ingredients:

- ✓ 2 tbsp olive oil, divided
- ✓ 1 large leek, white and light green parts, halved lengthwise, sliced ¼-inch thick
- ✓ 2 tsp chopped garlic
- ✓ 1 large red bell pepper, chopped into ¼-inch pieces
- ✓ 1 cup chopped fresh parsley leaves (1 small bunch)
- ✓ ½ cup chopped fresh cilantro leaves (½ small bunch)
- ✓ ¼ tsp ground cumin
- ✓ ¼ tsp ground coriander
- ✓ 1 tsp smoked paprika
- ✓ 1 pound uncooked peeled, deveined large shrimp (20 to 25 per pound), thawed if frozen, blotted with paper towels
- ✓ 1 tbsp freshly squeezed lemon juice
- ✓ ⅛ tsp kosher salt

Directions:

- ❖ Heat 2 tsp of oil in a -inch skillet over medium heat. Once the oil is hot, add the leeks and garlic and sauté for 2 minutes. Add the peppers and cook for 10 minutes, or until the peppers are soft, stirring occasionally.
- ❖ Add the chopped parsley and cilantro and cook for 1 more minute. Remove the mixture from the pan and place in a medium bowl.
- ❖ Mix the cumin, coriander, and paprika in a small prep bowl.
- ❖ Add 2 tsp of oil to the same skillet and increase the heat to medium-high. Add the shrimp in a single layer, sprinkle the spice mixture over the shrimp, and cook for about 2 minutes. Flip the shrimp over and cook for 1 more minute. Add the leek and herb mixture, stir, and cook for 1 more minute.
- ❖ Turn off the heat and add the remaining 2 tsp of oil and the lemon juice. Taste to see whether you need the salt. Add if necessary.
- ❖ Place ¾ cup of couscous or other grain (if using) and 1 cup of the shrimp mixture in each of 4 containers.
- ❖ STORAGE: Store covered containers in the refrigerator for up to 4 days.

69) Italian-style Chicken With Sweet Potato And Broccoli

	Cooking Time: 30 Minutes	Servings: 8

- ✓ 2 lbs boneless skinless chicken breasts, cut into small pieces
- ✓ 5-6 cups broccoli florets
- ✓ 3 tbsp Italian seasoning mix of your choice
- ✓ a few tbsp of olive oil
- ✓ 3 sweet potatoes, peeled and diced
- ✓ Coarse sea salt, to taste
- ✓ Freshly cracked pepper, to taste
- ✓ Toppings:
- ✓ Avocado
- ✓ Lemon juice
- ✓ Chives
- ✓ Olive oil, for serving

Directions:

- ❖ Preheat the oven to 425 degrees F
- ❖ Toss the chicken pieces with the Italian seasoning mix and a drizzle of olive oil, stir to combine then store in the fridge for about 30 minutes
- ❖ Arrange the broccoli florets and sweet potatoes on a sheet pan, drizzle with the olive oil, sprinkle generously with salt
- ❖ Arrange the chicken on a separate sheet pan
- ❖ Bake both in the oven for 12-1minutes
- ❖ Transfer the chicken and broccoli to a plate, toss the sweet potatoes and continue to roast for another 15 minutes, or until ready
- ❖ Allow the chicken, broccoli, and sweet potatoes to cool
- ❖ Distribute among the containers and store for 2-3 days
- ❖ To Serve: Reheat in the microwave for 1 minute or until heated through, top with the topping of choice. Enjoy
- ❖ Recipe Notes: Any kind of vegetables work will with this recipe! So, add favorites like carrots, brussels sprouts and asparagus.

Nutrition: Calories:222;Total Fat: 4.9g;Total Carbs: 15.3g;Protein: 28g

70) VEGETABLE SOUP

	Cooking Time: 20 Minutes	**Servings:** 6

Ingredients	Ingredients	Instructions
✓ 1 15-ounce can low sodium cannellini beans, drained and rinsed ✓ 1 tbsp olive oil ✓ 1 small onion, diced ✓ 2 carrots, diced ✓ 2 stalks celery, diced ✓ 1 small zucchini, diced ✓ 1 garlic clove, minced ✓ 1/3 cup freshly grated parmesan	✓ 1 tbsp fresh thyme leaves, chopped ✓ 2 tsp fresh sage, chopped ✓ ½ tsp salt ✓ ¼ tsp freshly ground black pepper ✓ 32 ounces low sodium chicken broth ✓ 1 14-ounce can no-salt diced tomatoes, undrained ✓ 2 cups baby spinach leaves, chopped	❖ Mash half of the beans in a small bowl using the back of a spoon and put it to the side. ❖ Add the oil to a large soup pot and place over medium-high heat. ❖ Add carrots, onion, celery, garlic, zucchini, thyme, salt, pepper, and sage. ❖ Cook well for about 5 minutes until the vegetables are tender. ❖ Add broth and tomatoes and bring the mixture to a boil. ❖ Add beans (both mashed and whole) and spinach. ❖ Cook for 3 minutes until the spinach has wilted. ❖ Pour the soup into the jars. ❖ Before serving, top with parmesan. ❖ Enjoy!

71) GREEK-STYLE CHICKEN WRAPS

	Cooking Time: 15 Minutes	**Servings:** 2

Ingredients	Ingredients	Instructions
✓ Greek Chicken Wrap Filling: ✓ 2 chicken breasts 14 oz, chopped into 1-inch pieces ✓ 2 small zucchinis, cut into 1-inch pieces ✓ 2 bell peppers, cut into 1-inch pieces ✓ 1 red onion, cut into 1-inch pieces ✓ 2 tbsp olive oil	✓ 2 tsp oregano ✓ 2 tsp basil ✓ 1/2 tsp garlic powder ✓ 1/2 tsp onion powder ✓ 1/2 tsp salt ✓ 2 lemons, sliced ✓ To Serve: ✓ 1/4 cup feta cheese crumbled ✓ 4 large flour tortillas or wraps	❖ Pre-heat oven to 425 degrees F ❖ In a bowl, toss together the chicken, zucchinis, olive oil, oregano, basil, garlic, bell peppers, onion powder, onion powder and salt ❖ Arrange lemon slice on the baking sheet(s), spread the chicken and vegetable out on top (use 2 baking sheets if needed) ❖ Bake for 15 minutes, until veggies are soft and the chicken is cooked through Allow to cool completely ❖ Distribute the chicken, bell pepper, zucchini and onions among the containers and remove the lemon slices Allow the dish to cool completely ❖ Distribute among the containers, store for 3 days ❖ To Serve: Reheat in the microwave for 1-2 minutes or until heated through. Wrap in a tortila and sprinkle with feta cheese. Enjoy

Nutrition: (1 wrap): Calories:356;Total Fat: 14g;Total Carbs: 26g;Protein: 29g

72) GARBANZO BEAN SOUP

	Cooking Time: 20 Minutes	**Servings:** 4

Ingredients	Ingredients	Instructions
✓ 14 ounces diced tomatoes ✓ 1 tsp olive oil ✓ 1 15-ounce can garbanzo beans	✓ salt ✓ pepper ✓ 2 sprigs fresh rosemary ✓ 1 cup acini di pepe pasta	❖ Take a large saucepan and add tomatoes and ounces of the beans. ❖ Bring the mixture to a boil over medium-high heat. ❖ Puree the remaining beans in a blender/food processor. ❖ Stir the pureed mixture into the pan. ❖ Add the sprigs of rosemary to the pan. ❖ Add acini de Pepe pasta and simmer until the pasta is soft, making sure to stir it from time to time. ❖ Remove the rosemary. ❖ Season with pepper and salt. ❖ Enjoy!

73) ITALIAN SALAD OF SPINACH AND BEANS

	Cooking Time: 30 Minutes	Servings: 4

✓ 15 ounces drained and rinsed cannellini beans ✓ 14 ounces drained, rinsed, and quartered artichoke hearts ✓ 6 ounces or 8 cups baby spinach ✓ 14 ½ ounces undrained diced tomatoes, no salt is best ✓ 1 tbsp olive oil and any additional if you prefer	✓ ¼ tsp salt ✓ 2 minced garlic cloves ✓ 1 chopped onion, small in size ✓ ¼ tsp pepper ✓ ⅛ tsp crushed red pepper flakes ✓ 2 tbsp Worcestershire sauce	❖ Place a saucepan on your stovetop and turn the temperature to medium-high. ❖ Let the pan warm up for a minute before you pour in the tbsp of oil. Continue to let the oil heat up for another minute or two. ❖ Toss in your chopped onion and stir so all the pieces are bathed in oil. Saute the onions for minutes. ❖ Add the garlic to the saucepan. Stir and saute the ingredients for another minute. ❖ Combine the salt, red pepper flakes, pepper, and Worcestershire sauce. Mix well and then add the tomatoes to the pan. Stir the mixture constantly for about minutes. ❖ Add the artichoke hearts, spinach, and beans. Saute and stir occasionally to get the taste throughout the dish. Once the spinach starts to wilt, take the salad off of the heat. ❖ Serve and enjoy immediately to get the best taste.

74) ITALIAN STYLE CHICKEN PASTA

	Cooking Time: 30 Minutes	Servings: 4

✓ Marinade: ✓ 1½ lbs. boneless, skinless chicken thighs, cut into bite-sized pieces* ✓ 2 garlic cloves, thinly sliced ✓ 2-3 tbsp. marinade from artichoke hearts ✓ 4 sprigs of fresh oregano, leaves stripped ✓ Olive oil ✓ Red wine vinegar ✓ Pasta: ✓ 1 lb whole wheat fusilli pasta ✓ 1 red onion, thinly sliced ✓ 1 pint grape or cherry tomatoes, whole	✓ ½ cup marinated artichoke hearts, roughly chopped ✓ ½ cup white beans, rinsed + drained (I use northern white beans) ✓ ½ cup Kalamata olives, roughly chopped ✓ ⅓ cup parsley and basil leaves, roughly chopped ✓ 2-3 handfuls of part-skim shredded mozzarella cheese ✓ Salt, to taste ✓ Pepper, to taste ✓ Garnish: ✓ Parsley ✓ Basil leaves	❖ Create the chicken marinade by drain the artichoke hearts reserving the juice ❖ In a large bowl, add the artichoke juice, garlic, chicken, and oregano leaves, drizzle with olive oil, a splash of red wine vinegar, and mix well to coat ❖ Marinate for at least 1 hour, maximum hours ❖ Cook the pasta in boiling salted water, drain and set aside ❖ Preheat your oven to 42degrees F ❖ In a casserole dish, add the sliced onions and tomatoes, toss with olive oil, salt and pepper. Then cook, stirring occasionally, until the onions are soft and the tomatoes start to burst, about 15-20 minutes ❖ In the meantime, in a large skillet over medium heat, add 1 tsp of olive oil ❖ Remove the chicken from the marinade, pat dry, and season with salt and pepper ❖ Working in batches, brown the chicken on both sides, leaving slightly undercooked ❖ Remove the casserole dish from the oven, add in the cooked pasta, browned chicken, artichoke hearts, beans, olives, and chopped herbs, stir to combine ❖ Top with grated cheese ❖ Bake for an additional 5-7 minutes, until the cheese is brown and bubbling ❖ Remove from the oven and allow the dish to cool completely ❖ Distribute among the containers, store for 2-3 days ❖ To Serve: Reheat in the microwave for 1-2 minutes or until heated through. ❖ Garnish with fresh herbs and serve

Nutrition: Calories:487;Carbs: 95g;Total Fat: 5g;Protein: 22g

75) FLAT BREAD WITH ROASTED VEGETABLES

	Cooking Time: 25 Minutes	Servings: 12

- 16 oz pizza dough, homemade or frozen
- 6 oz soft goat cheese, divided
- ¾ cup grated Parmesan cheese divided
- 3 tbsp chopped fresh dill, divided
- 1 small red onion, sliced thinly

- 1 small zucchini, sliced thinly
- 2 small tomatoes, thinly sliced
- 1 small red pepper, thinly sliced into rings
- Olive oil
- Salt, to taste
- Pepper, to taste

- Preheat the oven to 400 degrees F
- Roll the dough into a large rectangle, and then place it on a piece of parchment paper sprayed with non-stick spray
- Take a knife and spread half the goat cheese onto one half of the dough, then sprinkle with half the dill and half the Parmesan cheese
- Carefully fold the other half of the dough on top of the cheese, spread and sprinkle the remaining parmesan and goat cheese
- Layer the thinly sliced vegetables over the top
- Brush the olive oil over the top of the veggies and sprinkle with salt, pepper, and the remaining dill
- Bake for 22-25 minutes, until the edges are medium brown, cut in half, lengthwise
- Then slice the flatbread in long 2-inch slices and allow to cool
- Distribute among the containers, store for 2 days
- To Serve: Reheat in the oven at 375 degrees for 5 minutes or until hot. Enjoy with a fresh salad.

76) COBB SALAD WITH STEAK

	Cooking Time: 15 Minutes	Servings: 4

- 6 large eggs
- 2 tbsp unsalted butter
- 1 lb steak
- 2 tbsp olive oil
- 6 cups baby spinach

- 1 cup cherry tomatoes, halved
- 1 cup pecan halves
- 1/2 cup crumbled feta cheese
- Kosher salt, to taste
- Freshly ground black pepper, to taste

- In a large skillet over medium high heat, melt butter
- Using paper towels, pat the steak dry, then drizzle with olive oil and season with salt and pepper, to taste
- Once heated, add the steak to the skillet and cook, flipping once, until cooked through to desired doneness, - cook for 4 minutes per side for a medium-rare steak
- Transfer the steak to a plate and allow it to cool before dicing Place the eggs in a large saucepan and cover with cold water by 1 inch
- Bring to a boil and cook for 1 minute, cover the eggs with a tight-fitting lid and remove from heat, set aside for 8-10 minutes, then drain well and allow to cool before peeling and dicing Assemble the salad in the container by placing the spinach at the bottom of the container, top with arranged rows of steak, eggs, feta, tomatoes, and pecans
- To Serve: Top with the balsamic vinaigrette, or desired dressing

77) LAMB CHOPS GRILL

	Cooking Time: 10 Minutes	Servings: 4

- 4 8-ounce lamb shoulder chops
- 2 tbsp Dijon mustard
- 2 tbsp balsamic vinegar

- 1 tbsp chopped garlic
- ¼ tsp ground black pepper
- ½ cup olive oil
- 2 tbsp fresh basil, shredded

- Pat the lamb chops dry and arrange them in a shallow glass-baking dish.
- Take a bowl and whisk in Dijon mustard, garlic, balsamic vinegar, and pepper. Mix well to make the marinade.
- Whisk oil slowly into the marinade until it is smooth.
- Stir in basil. Pour the marinade over the lamb chops, making sure to coat both sides.
- Cover, refrigerate and allow the chops to marinate for anywhere from 1-4 hours. Remove the chops from the refrigerator and leave out for 30 minutes or until room temperature.
- Preheat grill to medium heat and oil grate.
- Grill the lamb chops until the center reads 145 degrees F and they are nicely browned, about 5-minutes per side.
- Enjoy!

78) CHILI BROILED SQUID

Cooking Time: 8 Minutes	Servings: 4

✓ 2 tbsp extra virgin olive oil ✓ 1 tsp chili powder ✓ ½ tsp ground cumin ✓ Zest of 1 lime ✓ Juice of 1 lime	✓ Dash of sea salt ✓ 1 and ½ pounds squid, cleaned and split open, with tentacles cut into ½ inch rounds ✓ 2 tbsp cilantro, chopped ✓ 2 tbsp red bell pepper, minced	❖ Take a medium bowl and stir in olive oil, chili powder, cumin, lime zest, sea salt, lime juice and pepper ❖ Add squid and let it marinade and stir to coat, coat and let it refrigerate for 1 hour ❖ Pre-heat your oven to broil ❖ Arrange squid on a baking sheet, broil for 8 minutes turn once until tender ❖ Garnish the broiled calamari with cilantro and red bell pepper ❖ Serve and enjoy! ❖ Meal Prep/Storage Options: Store in airtight containers in your fridge for 1-2 days.

Nutrition: Calories:159;Fat: 13g;Carbohydrates: 12g;Protein: 3g

79) SALMON AND CORN BELL PEPPER SAUCE

Cooking Time: 12 Minutes	Servings: 2

✓ 1 garlic clove, grated ✓ ½ tsp mild chili powder ✓ ½ tsp ground coriander ✓ ¼ tsp ground cumin ✓ 2 limes – 1, zest and juice; 1 cut into wedges ✓ 2 tsp rapeseed oil	✓ 2 wild salmon fillets ✓ 1 ear of corn on the cob, husk removed ✓ 1 red onion, finely chopped ✓ 1 avocado, cored, peeled, and finely chopped ✓ 1 red pepper, deseeded and finely chopped ✓ 1 red chili, halved and deseeded ✓ ½ a pack of finely chopped coriander	❖ Boil the corn in water for about 6-8 minutes until tender. ❖ Drain and cut off the kernels. ❖ In a bowl, combine garlic, spices, 1 tbsp of limejuice, and oil; mix well to prepare spice rub. ❖ Coat the salmon with the rub. ❖ Add the zest to the corn and give it a gentle stir. ❖ Heat a frying pan over medium heat. ❖ Add salmon and cook for about 2 minutes per side. ❖ Serve the cooked salmon with salsa and lime wedges. ❖ Enjoy!

80) ITALIAN-INSPIRED ROTISSERIE CHICKEN WITH BROCCOLI SLAW

Cooking Time: 15 Minutes	Servings: 4

✓ 4 cups packaged broccoli slaw ✓ 1 cooked rotisserie chicken, meat removed (about 10 to 12 ounces) ✓ 1 bunch red radishes, stemmed, halved, and thickly sliced (about 1¼ cups) ✓ 1 cup sliced red onion	✓ ½ cup pitted kalamata or niçoise olives, roughly chopped ✓ ½ cup sliced pepperoncini ✓ 8 tbsp Dijon Red Wine Vinaigrette, divided	❖ Place the broccoli slaw, chicken, radishes, onion, olives, and pepperoncini in a large mixing bowl. Toss to combine. ❖ Place cups of salad in each of 4 containers. Pour 2 tbsp of vinaigrette into each of 4 sauce containers. ❖ STORAGE: Store covered containers in the refrigerator for up to 5 days.

Nutrition: Total calories: 329; Total fat: 2; Saturated fat: 4g; Sodium: 849mg; Carbohydrates: 10g; Fiber: 3g; Protein: 20g

81) FLATBREAD AND ROASTED VEGETABLES

Cooking Time: 45 Minutes	Servings: 12

Ingredients:

- ✓ 5 ounces goat cheese
- ✓ 1 thinly sliced onion
- ✓ 2 thinly sliced tomatoes
- ✓ Olive oil
- ✓ ¼ tsp pepper
- ✓ ⅛ tsp salt
- ✓ 16 ounces homemade or frozen pizza dough
- ✓ ¾ tbsp chopped dill, fresh is better
- ✓ 1 thinly sliced zucchini
- ✓ 1 red pepper, cup into rings

❖ Set your oven to 400 degrees Fahrenheit.

❖ Set the dough on a large piece of parchment paper. Use a rolling pin to roll the dough into a large rectangle.

❖ Spread half of the goat cheese on ½ of the pizza dough.

❖ Sprinkle half of the dill on the other half of the dough.

❖ Fold the dough so the half with the dill is on top of the cheese.

❖ Spread the remaining goat cheese on the pizza dough and then sprinkle the rest of the dill over the cheese.

❖ Layer the vegetables on top in any arrangement you like.

❖ Drizzle olive oil on top of the vegetables.

❖ Sprinkle salt and pepper over the olive oil.

❖ Set the piece of parchment paper on a pizza pan or baking pan and place it in the oven.

❖ Set the timer for 22 minutes. If the edges are not a medium brown, leave the flatbread in the oven for another couple of minutes.

❖ Remove the pizza from the oven when it is done and cut the flatbread in half lengthwise.

❖ Slice the flatbread into 2-inch long pieces and enjoy!

Nutrition: calories: 170, fats: 5 grams, carbohydrates: 20 grams, protein: 8 grams.

82) SEAFOOD RICE

Cooking Time: 40 Minutes	Servings: 4-5

- ✓ 4 small lobster tails (6-12 oz each)
- ✓ Water
- ✓ 3 tbsp Extra Virgin Olive Oil
- ✓ 1 large yellow onion, chopped
- ✓ 2 cups Spanish rice or short grain rice, soaked in water for 15 minutes and then drained
- ✓ 4 garlic cloves, chopped
- ✓ 2 large pinches of Spanish saffron threads soaked in 1/2 cup water
- ✓ 1 tsp Sweet Spanish paprika
- ✓ 1 tsp cayenne pepper
- ✓ 1/2 tsp aleppo pepper flakes
- ✓ Salt, to taste
- ✓ 2 large Roma tomatoes, finely chopped
- ✓ 6 oz French green beans, trimmed
- ✓ 1 lb prawns or large shrimp or your choice, peeled and deveined
- ✓ 1/4 cup chopped fresh parsley

❖ In a large pot, add 3 cups of water and bring it to a rolling boil

❖ Add in the lobster tails and allow boil briefly, about 1-minutes or until pink, remove from heat

❖ Using tongs transfer the lobster tails to a plate and Do not discard the lobster cooking water

❖ Allow the lobster is cool, then remove the shell and cut into large chunks.

❖ In a large deep pan or skillet over medium-high heat, add 3 tbsp olive oil

❖ Add the chopped onions, sauté the onions for 2 minutes and then add the rice, and cook for 3 more minutes, stirring regularly

❖ Then add in the lobster cooking water and the chopped garlic and, stir in the saffron and its soaking liquid, cayenne pepper, aleppo pepper, paprika, and salt

❖ Gently stir in the chopped tomatoes and green beans, bring to a boil and allow the liquid slightly reduce, then cover (with lid or tightly wrapped foil) and cook over low heat for 20 minutes

❖ Once done, uncover and spread the shrimp over the rice, push it into the rice slightly, add in a little water, if needed

❖ Cover and cook for another 15 minutes until the shrimp turn pink

❖ Then add in the cooked lobster chunks

❖ Once the lobster is warmed through, remove from heat allow the dish to cool completely

❖ Distribute among the containers, store for 2 days

❖ To Serve: Reheat in the microwave for 1-2 minutes or until heated through. Garnish with parsley and enjoy!

❖ Recipe Notes: Remember to soak your rice if needed to help with the cooking process

Nutrition: Calories:536;Carbs: 56g;Total Fat: 26g;Protein: 50g

83) ITALIAN STYLE PEARL COUSCOUS

Cooking Time: 10 Minutes		Servings: 6

✓ For the Lemon Dill Vinaigrette: ✓ 1 large lemon, juice of ✓ 1/3 cup Extra virgin olive oil ✓ 1 tsp dill weed ✓ 1 tsp garlic powder ✓ Salt and pepper ✓ For the Israeli Couscous: ✓ 2 cups Pearl Couscous, Israeli Couscous ✓ Extra virgin olive oil	✓ 2 cups grape tomatoes, halved ✓ 1/3 cup finely chopped red onions ✓ 1/2 English cucumber, finely chopped ✓ 15 oz can chickpeas ✓ 14 oz can good quality artichoke hearts, roughly chopped if needed ✓ 1/2 cup good pitted kalamata olives ✓ 15–20 fresh basil leaves, roughly chopped or torn; more for garnish ✓ 3 oz fresh baby mozzarella or feta cheese, optional ✓ Water

❖ Make the lemon-dill vinaigrette, place the lemon juice, olive oil, dill weed, garlic powder, salt and pepper in a bowl, whisk together to combine and set aside

❖ In a medium-sized heavy pot, heat two tbsp of olive oil

❖ Sauté the couscous in the olive oil briefly until golden brown, then add cups of boiling water (or follow the instructed on the package), and cook according to package.

❖ Once done, drain in a colander, set aside in a bowl and allow to cool

❖ In a large mixing bowl, combine the extra virgin olive oil, grape tomatoes, red onions, cucumber, chickpeas, artichoke hearts, and kalamata olives

❖ Then add in the couscous and the basil, mix together gently

❖ Now, give the lemon-dill vinaigrette a quick whisk and add to the couscous salad, mix to combine

❖ Taste and adjust salt, if needed

❖ Distribute among the containers, store for 2-3 days

❖ To Serve: Add in the mozzarella cheese, garnish with more fresh basil and enjoy

Nutrition: Calories:393;Carbs: 57g;Total Fat: 13g;Protein: 13g

84) POTATOES WITH TUNA SALAD

Cooking Time: Nil		Servings: 4

✓ 1-pound baby potatoes, scrubbed, boiled ✓ 1 cup tuna chunks, drained ✓ 1 cup cherry tomatoes, halved ✓ 1 cup medium onion, thinly sliced ✓ 8 pitted black olives ✓ 2 medium hard-boiled eggs, sliced	✓ 1 head Romaine lettuce ✓ Honey lemon mustard dressing ✓ ¼ cup olive oil ✓ 2 tbsp lemon juice ✓ 1 tbsp Dijon mustard ✓ 1 tsp dill weed, chopped ✓ Salt as needed ✓ Pepper as needed

❖ Take a small glass bowl and mix in your olive oil, honey, lemon juice, Dijon mustard and dill

❖ Season the mix with pepper and salt

❖ Add in the tuna, baby potatoes, cherry tomatoes, red onion, green beans, black olives and toss everything nicely

❖ Arrange your lettuce leaves on a beautiful serving dish to make the base of your salad

❖ Top them up with your salad mixture and place the egg slices

❖ Drizzle it with the previously prepared Salad Dressing

❖ Serve hot

❖ Meal Prep/Storage Options: Store in airtight containers in your fridge for 1-2 days. Keep the fish and salad ingredients separated, mix together before serving!

Nutrition: Calories: 406;Fat: 22g;Carbohydrates: 28g;Protein: 26g

85) EGGPLANT STUFFED WITH QUINOA AND TAHINI SAUCE

	Cooking Time: 30 Minutes	Servings: 2

✓ 1 eggplant
✓ 2 tbsp olive oil, divided
✓ 1 medium shallot, diced, about 1/2 cup
✓ 1 cup chopped button mushrooms, about 2 cups whole
✓ 5-6 Tuttorosso whole plum tomatoes, chopped
✓ 1 tbsp tomato juice from the can
✓ 1 tbsp chopped fresh parsley, plus more to garnish

✓ 2 garlic cloves, minced
✓ 1/2 cup cooked quinoa
✓ 1/2 tsp ground cumin
✓ Salt, to taste
✓ Pepper, to taste
✓ 1 tbsp tahini
✓ 1 tsp lemon juice
✓ 1/2 tsp garlic powder
✓ Water to thin

❖ Preheat the oven to 425 degrees F
❖ Prepare the eggplant by cutting it in half lengthwise and scoop out some of the flesh
❖ Place it on a baking sheet, drizzle with 1 tbsp of oil, sprinkle with salt
❖ Bake for 20 minutes
❖ In the meantime, add the remaining oil in a large skillet
❖ Once heated, add the shallots and mushrooms, sauté until mushrooms have softened, about 5 minutes Add in the tomatoes, quinoa and spices, cook until the liquid has evaporated
❖ Once the eggplant has cooked, reduce the oven temperature to 350 degrees F
❖ Stuff each half with the tomato-quinoa mixture
❖ Bake for another 10 minutes
❖ Allow to cool completely
❖ Distribute among the containers, store for 2 days
❖ To Serve: Reheat in the microwave for 1-2 minutes or until heated through. Quickly whisk together tahini, lemon, garlic, water and a sprinkle of salt and pepper, drizzle tahini over eggplants and sprinkle with parsley and enjoy.

Nutrition: Calories:345;Carbs: 38g;Total Fat: 19g;Protein: 9g

86) ITALIAN-STYLE LASAGNA

	Cooking Time: 1 Hour 15 Minutes	Servings: 8

✓ Lasagna noodles, oven-ready are the best, easiest, and quickest
✓ ⅓ cup flour
✓ 2 tbsp chives, divided and chopped
✓ ½ cup white wine
✓ 2 tbsp olive oil
✓ 1 ½ tbsp thyme
✓ 1 tsp salt
✓ 1 ¼ cups shallots, chopped
✓ 1 cup boiled water
✓ ½ cup Parmigiano-Reggiano cheese

✓ 3 cups milk, reduced-fat and divided
✓ 1 tbsp butter
✓ ⅓ cup cream cheese, less fat is the best choice
✓ 6 cloves of garlic, divided and minced
✓ ½ tsp ground black pepper, divided
✓ 4 ounces dried shiitake mushrooms, sliced
✓ 1 ounce dried porcini mushrooms, sliced
✓ 8 ounces cremini mushrooms, sliced

❖ Keeping your mushrooms separated, drain them all and return them to separate containers.
❖ Bring 1 cup of water to a boil and cook your porcini mushrooms for a half hour.
❖ Preheat your oven to 0 degrees Fahrenheit.
❖ Set a large pan on your stove and turn the burner to medium-high heat.
❖ Add your butter and let it melt.
❖ Combine the olive oil and shallots. Stir the mixture and let it cook for 3 minutes.
❖ Pour half of the pepper, half of the salt, and mushrooms into the pan. Allow the mixture to cook for 6 minutes.
❖ While stirring, add half of the garlic and thyme. Continue to stir for 1 minute.
❖ Pour the wine and turn your burner temperature to high. Let the mixture boil and watch the liquid evaporate for a couple of minutes to reduce it slightly.
❖ Turn off the burner and remove the pan from heat.
❖ Add the cream cheese and chives. Stir thoroughly.
❖ Set a medium-sized skillet on medium-high heat and add 1 tbsp of oil. Let the oil come to a simmer.
❖ Add the last of the garlic to the pan and saute for 30 seconds.
❖ Pour in 2 ⅓ cup milk and the liquid from the porcini mushrooms. Stir the mixture and allow it to boil.
❖ In a bowl, combine ¼ cup of milk and the flour. Add this mixture to the heated pan. Stir until the mixture starts to thicken.
❖ Grease a pan and add ½ cup of sauce along with a row of noodles.
❖ Spread half of the mushroom mixture on top of the noodles.
❖ Repeat the process, but make sure you top the lasagna with mushrooms and cheese.
❖ Turn your timer to 45 minutes and set the pan into the oven.
❖ Remember to garnish the lasagna with chives before enjoying!

Nutrition: calories: 268, fats: 12.6 grams, carbohydrates: 29 grams, protein: 10 grams.

87) TUNA AND VEGETABLE MIX

		Cooking Time: 15 Minutes	Servings: 4

✓ ¼ cup extra-virgin olive oil, divided ✓ 1 tbsp rice vinegar ✓ 1 tsp kosher salt, divided ✓ ¾ tsp Dijon mustard ✓ ¾ tsp honey ✓ 4 ounces baby gold beets, thinly sliced	✓ 4 ounces fennel bulb, trimmed and thinly sliced ✓ 4 ounces baby turnips, thinly sliced ✓ 6 ounces Granny Smith apple, very thinly sliced ✓ 2 tsp sesame seeds, toasted ✓ 6 ounces tuna steaks ✓ ½ tsp black pepper ✓ 1 tbsp fennel fronds, torn	❖ In a large bowl, add 2 tbsp of oil, ½ a tsp of salt, honey, vinegar, and mustard. ❖ Give the mixture a nice mix. ❖ Add fennel, beets, apple, and turnips; mix and toss until everything is evenly coated. ❖ Sprinkle with sesame seeds and toss well. ❖ In a cast-iron skillet, heat 2 tbsp of oil over high heat. ❖ Carefully season the tuna with ½ a tsp of salt and pepper ❖ Place the tuna in the skillet and cook for about 3 minutes total, giving 1½ minutes per side. ❖ Remove the tuna and slice it up. ❖ Place in containers with the vegetable mix. ❖ Serve with the fennel mix, and enjoy!

88) SPICY BURGERS

		Cooking Time: 25-30 Minutes	Servings: 6/2 Chops Each

✓ Medium onion (1) ✓ Fresh parsley (3 tbsp.) ✓ Clove of garlic (1) ✓ Ground allspice (.75 tsp.) ✓ Pepper (.75 tsp.) ✓ Ground nutmeg (.25 tsp.)	✓ Cinnamon (.5 tsp.) ✓ Salt (.5 tsp.) ✓ Fresh mint (2 tbsp.) ✓ 90% lean ground beef (1.5 lb.) ✓ Optional: Cold Tzatziki sauce	❖ Finely chop/mince the parsley, mint, garlic, and onions. ❖ Whisk the nutmeg, salt, cinnamon, pepper, allspice, garlic, mint, parsley, and onion. ❖ Add the beef and prepare six (6 2x4-inch oblong patties. ❖ Use the medium temperature setting to grill the patties or broil them four inches from the heat source for four to six minutes per side. ❖ When they're done, the meat thermometer will register 160° Fahrenheit. Serve with the sauce if desired.

89) TUNA AND CABBAGE BOWL

		Cooking Time: 15 To 20 Minutes	Servings: 6

✓ 3 tbsp extra virgin olive oil ✓ 1 ½ tsp minced garlic ✓ ¼ cup of capers ✓ 2 tsp sugar ✓ 15 ounce can of drained and rinsed great northern beans ✓ 1 pound chopped kale with the center ribs removed	✓ ½ tsp ground black pepper ✓ 1 cup chopped onion ✓ 2 ½ ounces of drained sliced olives ✓ ¼ tsp sea salt ✓ ¼ tsp crushed red pepper ✓ 6 ounces of tuna in olive oil, do not drain	❖ Place a large pot, like a stockpot, on your stove and turn the burner to high heat. ❖ Fill the pot about 3-quarters of the way full with water and let it come to a boil. ❖ Add the kale and cook for 2 minutes. ❖ Drain the kale and set it aside. ❖ Turn the heat down to medium and place the empty pot back on the burner. ❖ Add the oil and onion. Saute for 3 to 4 minutes. ❖ Combine the garlic into the oil mixture and saute for another minute. ❖ Add the capers, olives, and red pepper. ❖ Cook the ingredients for another minute while stirring. ❖ Pour in the sugar and stir while you toss in the kale. Mix all the ingredients thoroughly and ensure the kale is thoroughly coated. ❖ Cover the pot and set the timer for 8 minutes. ❖ Turn off the heat and add in the tuna, pepper, beans, salt, and any other herbs that will make this one of the best Italian -Style dishes you've ever made.

90) POMODORO SOUP

	Cooking Time: 30 Minutes	Servings: 8

Ingredients	More Ingredients	Instructions
✓ 4 tbsp olive oil ✓ 2 medium yellow onions, thinly sliced ✓ 1 tsp salt (extra for taste if needed) ✓ 2 tsp curry powder ✓ 1 tsp red curry powder ✓ 1 tsp ground coriander ✓ ¼-½ tsp red pepper flakes ✓	✓ 1 15-ounce can diced tomatoes, undrained ✓ 1 28-ounce can diced or plum tomatoes, undrained ✓ 5½ cups water (vegetable broth or chicken broth also usable) ✓ 1 14-ounce can coconut milk ✓ optional add-ins: cooked brown rice, lemon wedges, fresh thyme, etc.	❖ Heat oil in a medium-sized pot over medium heat. ❖ Add onions and salt and cook for about 10-1minutes until browned. ❖ Stir in curry powder, coriander, red pepper flakes, cumin, and cook for seconds, being sure to keep stirring well. ❖ Add tomatoes and water (or broth if you prefer). ❖ Simmer the mixture for 1minutes. ❖ Take an immersion blender and puree the mixture until a soupy consistency is achieved. ❖ Enjoy as it is, or add some extra add-ins for a more flavorful experience

91) ONION AND CHEESE SOUP

	Cooking Time: 25 Minutes	Servings: 4

Ingredients	More Ingredients	Instructions
✓ 2 large onions, finely sliced ✓ 2 cups vegetable stock ✓ 1 tsp brown sugar ✓ 1 cup red wine ✓ 1 measure of brandy ✓ 1 tsp herbs de Provence	✓ 4 slices stale bread ✓ 4 ounces grated strong cheese ✓ 1-ounce grated parmesan ✓ 1 tbsp plain flour ✓ 2 tbsp olive oil ✓ 1-ounce butter ✓ salt ✓ pepper	❖ Heat oil and butter in a pan over medium-high heat. ❖ Add onions and brown sugar. ❖ Cook until the onions are golden brown. ❖ Pour brandy and flambé, making sure to keep stirring until the flames are out. ❖ Add plain flour and herbs de Provence and keep stirring well. ❖ Slowly add the stock and red wine. ❖ Season well and simmer for 20 minutes, making sure to add water if the soup becomes too thick. ❖ Ladle the soup into jars. ❖ Before serving, place rounds of stale bread on top. ❖ Add strong cheese. ❖ Garnish with some parmesan. ❖ Place the bowls under a hot grill or in an oven until the cheese has melted.

92) ITALIAN STYLE SNAPPER

	Cooking Time: 12 Minutes	Servings: 4

Ingredients	More Ingredients	Instructions
✓ non-stick cooking spray ✓ 2 tbsp extra virgin olive oil ✓ 1 medium onion, chopped ✓ 2 garlic cloves, minced ✓ 1 tsp oregano ✓ 1 14-ounce can diced tomatoes, undrained	✓ ½ cup black olives, sliced ✓ 4 4-ounce red snapper fillets ✓ salt ✓ pepper ✓ ¼ cup crumbled feta cheese ✓ ¼ cup fresh parsley, minced	❖ Preheat oven to 425 degrees Fahrenheit. ❖ Grease a 13x9 baking dish with non-stick cooking spray. ❖ Heat oil in a large skillet over medium heat. ❖ Add onion, oregano, garlic, and sauté for 2 minutes. ❖ Add can of tomatoes and olives, and bring mixture to a boil; remove from heat. ❖ Season both sides of fillets with salt and pepper and place in the baking dish. ❖ Spoon the tomato mixture evenly over the fish. ❖ Bake for 10 minutes. ❖ Remove from oven and sprinkle with parsley and feta. ❖ Enjoy!

93) PAN-FRIED ITALIAN CHICKEN AND MUSHROOMS WITH TOMATOES

Cooking Time: 20 Minutes		Servings: 4

✓ 4 large chicken cutlets, boneless skinless chicken breasts cut into 1/4-inch thin cutlets
✓ 1 tbsp dried oregano, divided
✓ 1/2 cup all-purpose flour, more for later
✓ 8 oz Baby Bella mushrooms, cleaned, trimmed, and sliced
✓ 14 oz grape tomatoes, halved
✓ 2 tbsp chopped fresh garlic

✓ Extra Virgin Olive Oil
✓ 1/2 cup white wine
✓ 1 tbsp freshly squeezed lemon juice, juice of 1/2 lemon
✓ 1 tsp salt, divided
✓ 1 tsp black pepper, divided
✓ 3/4 cup chicken broth
✓ Handful baby spinach, optional

❖ Pat the chicken cutlets dry, season both sides with 2 tsp salt, 1/2 tsp black pepper, 1/2 tbsp dried oregano,
❖ Coat the chicken cutlets with the flour, gently dust-off excess and set aside
❖ In a large cast iron skillet with a lid, heat 2 tbsp olive oil
❖ Once heated, brown the chicken cutlets on both sides, for about 3 minutes, then transfer the chicken cutlets to plate
❖ In the same skillet, add more olive oil if needed,
❖ Once heated, add in the mushrooms and sauté on medium-high for about 1 minute
❖ Then add the tomatoes, garlic, the remaining 1/2 tbsp oregano, 1/2 tsp salt, and 1/2 tsp pepper, and 2 tsp flour, cook for 3 minutes or so, stirring regularly
❖ Add in the white wine, cook briefly to reduce, then add the lemon juice and chicken broth
❖ Bring the liquid to a boil, then transfer the chicken back into the skillet, cook over high heat for 3-4 minutes, then reduce the heat to medium-low, cover and cook for another 8 minutes or until the chicken is cooked through
❖ Allow the dish to cool completely
❖ Distribute among the containers, store for 3 days
❖ To Serve: Reheat in the microwave for 1-2 minutes or until heated through. Serve with baby spinach, your favorite small pasta and a crusty Italian bread!

94) ROAST BRAISED IN RED WINE AND CARROTS WITH MUSHROOMS

Cooking Time: 25 Minutes		Servings: 4

Ingredients:

✓ 1 pound tri-tip roast
✓ ¼ tsp kosher salt
✓ 1 tbsp olive oil
✓ 2 cups chopped onion
✓ 1 tsp chopped garlic
✓ 3 medium carrots, cut into ½-inch pieces (2 cups)
✓ 2 large celery stalks, cut into ½-inch pieces (1 cup)

✓ 8 ounces button or cremini mushrooms, halved
✓ ½ tsp fennel seed
✓ ½ tsp dried thyme
✓ ½ tsp dried oregano
✓ 1 (14.5-ounce) can no-salt-added diced tomatoes
✓ 1 cup dry red wine, such as red zinfandel or cabernet sauvignon
✓ 1 cup reduced-sodium beef broth

Directions:

❖ Preheat the oven to 325°F.
❖ Season the roast with the salt.
❖ Heat the oil in a Dutch oven or heavy-bottomed soup pot over high heat. Once the oil is hot, add the roast and brown for minutes on each side. Remove the roast to a plate.
❖ Add the onion, garlic, carrots, celery, and mushrooms to the pot and cook for 5 minutes.
❖ Add the fennel seed, thyme, oregano, tomatoes, red wine, and broth and bring to a simmer. Cover the pot with a tight-fitting lid or foil and place in the oven. Cook until the meat is very tender, about 3 hours.
❖ Remove the roast to a plate and spoon the vegetables into a bowl with a slotted spoon. Place the pot on high heat and reduce the liquid by half, about 10 minutes. If your pot is extra wide, it will take less time for the liquid to reduce. Add more salt if needed.
❖ After the meat has cooled, cut 12 slices against the grain. Place 3 slices, ¾ cup of vegetables, and ⅓ cup of sauce in each of 4 containers.
❖ STORAGE: Store covered containers in the refrigerator for up to 5 days.

Nutrition: Total calories: 366; Total fat: 14g; Saturated fat: 4g; Sodium: 468mg; Carbohydrates: 23g; Fiber: 6g; Protein: 28g

95) ZOODLES AND TURKEY MEATBALLS

	Cooking Time: 30 Minutes	Servings: 4-6

✓ 2 lbs (3 medium-sized) zucchini, spiralized ✓ 2 cups marinara sauce, store-bought ✓ 1/4 cup freshly grated Parmesan cheese ✓ 2 tsp salt ✓ For The Meatballs: ✓ 1 ½ lbs ground turkey ✓ 1/2 cup Panko	✓ 1/4 cup freshly grated Parmesan cheese ✓ 2 large egg yolks ✓ 1 tsp dried oregano ✓ 1 tsp dried basil ✓ 1/2 tsp dried parsley ✓ 1/4 tsp garlic powder ✓ 1/4 tsp crushed red pepper flakes ✓ Kosher salt, to taste ✓ Freshly ground black pepper, to taste	❖ Preheat oven to 400 degrees F ❖ Lightly oil a 9×13 baking dish or spray with nonstick spray ❖ In a large bowl, combine the ground turkey, egg yolks, oregano, basil, Panko, Parmesan, parsley, garlic powder and red pepper flakes, season the mixture with salt and pepper, to taste ❖ Use a wooden spoon or clean hands, stir well to combined ❖ Roll the mixture into 1 1/2-to-2-inch meatballs, forming about 24 meatballs ❖ Place the meatballs onto the prepared baking dish ❖ Bake for 18-20 minutes, or until browned and the meatballs are cooked through, set aside ❖ Place the zucchini in a colander over the sink, add the salt and gently toss to combine, allow to sit for 10 minutes ❖ In a large pot of boiling water, cook zucchini for 30 seconds to 1 minute, drain well ❖ Allow to cool, then distribute the zucchini into the containers, top with the meatballs, marinara sauce and the Parmesan. Store in the fridge for up to 4 days ❖ To Serve: Reheat in the microwave for 1-2 minutes or until heated through and enjoy!

96) ENGLISH PLATTER

	Cooking Time: 45 Minutes	Servings: 2

✓ 1 garlic clove, minced ✓ 5-ounce fresh button mushrooms, sliced ✓ 1/8 cup unsalted butter ✓ ¼ tsp dried thyme	✓ 1/3 cup heavy whipping cream ✓ Salt and black pepper, to taste ✓ 2 (6-ounce grass-fed New York strip steaks	❖ Preheat the grill to medium heat and grease it. ❖ Season the steaks with salt and black pepper, and transfer to the grill. ❖ Grill steaks for about 10 minutes on each side and dish out in a platter. ❖ Put butter, mushrooms, salt and black pepper in a pan and cook for about 10 minutes. ❖ Add thyme and garlic and thyme and sauté for about 1 minute. ❖ Stir in the cream and let it simmer for about 5 minutes. ❖ Top the steaks with mushroom sauce and serve hot immediately. ❖ Meal Prep Tip: You can store the mushroom sauce in refrigerator for about 2 days. Season the steaks carefully with salt and black pepper to avoid low or high quantities.

97) ITALIAN -STYLE PIZZA

	Cooking Time: 20 Minutes	Servings: 4 To 8

✓ 1/2 cup artichoke hearts ✓ Whole-wheat premade pizza crust ✓ 1 cup pesto sauce ✓ 1 cup spinach leaves ✓ 3 to 4 ounces of feta cheese	✓ 1 cup sun-dried tomatoes ✓ 3 ounces of mozzarella cheese ✓ ½ cup of olives ✓ Olive oil ✓ ½ cup bell peppers ✓ Chopped chicken, pepperoni, or salami	❖ Turn the temperature of your oven to 350 degrees Fahrenheit. ❖ Use olive oil to brush the top of the whole wheat pizza crust. ❖ Brush the pesto sauce on the pizza crust. ❖ Top with all of the ingredients. You can start with the cheese or mix the ingredients in any way you wish. You can even get a little creative and have fun. ❖ Set your pizza on a pizza pan or directly on your oven rack. ❖ Set your timer to 10 minutes, but watch the pizza carefully so you do not burn the cheese. ❖ Remove the pizza and let it cool down for a couple of minutes, then enjoy!

98) SALMON TZATZIKI BOWL GRILL

	Cooking Time: 15 Minutes	Servings: 2

✓ 8–10 ounces salmon, serves 2 ✓ Olive oil for brushing ✓ Salt and pepper ✓ 1 lemon- sliced in half ✓ Tzatziki: ✓ ½ cup plain yogurt ✓ ½ cup sour cream ✓ 1 garlic clove- finely minced ✓ 1 tbsp lemon juice, more to taste ✓ 1 tbsp olive oil ✓ ½ tsp kosher salt ✓ ¼ tsp white pepper or black ✓ ⅛ cup fresh chopped dill (or mint, cilantro or Italian parsley – or a mix)	✓ 1 ½ cups finely sliced or diced cucumber ✓ Optional Bowl Additions: ✓ Cooked Quinoa or rice ✓ Arugula or other greens ✓ Grilled veggies like eggplant, peppers, tomatoes, or zucchini ✓ Fresh veggies of your choice - radishes, cucumber, tomatoes, sprouts ✓ Garnish with olive oil, lemon, and fresh herbs	❖ Preheat heat grill to medium high ❖ Cook 1 cup quinoa or rice on the stove, according to directions, allow to cool ❖ Brush the salmon with olive oil, season with salt and pepper, set aside ❖ Create the Tzatziki, by adding plain yogurt, sour cream, garlic clove, lemon juice, olive oil, kosher salt, and white pepper in a bowl, taste and add more lemon juice if desired, store in fridge ❖ Place the salmon on the grill, along with the veggies of you choose to grill, brushing all with olive oil, salt and pepper ❖ Grill the salmon on both sides for 3-4 minutes, or until cooked through ❖ Then grill the lemon, open side down, until good grill marks appear ❖ Once the veggies and salmon are done, allow them to cool ❖ Distribute among the containers - Divide quinoa among the containers, arrange the grilled vegetables and salmon over top. ❖ To Serve: Reheat in the microwave for 1 minute or until heated through. Top with the greens and the fresh veggies, then drizzle a little olive oil on top and season with salt, squeeze the grilled lemon over the whole bowl, spoon the tzatziki over top the salmon, sprinkle with the fresh dill or other herbs. Enjoy with a glass of wine.

Nutrition: Calories:458;Carbs: 29g;Total Fat: 24g;Protein: 30g

99) BUTTERNUT SMOKED BEET, CHICKPEA AND PUMPKIN SOUP

	Cooking Time: 35 Minutes	Servings: 8

✓ 2 slices bacon (about 1 ounce), chopped ✓ 1 cup chopped onion ✓ 1 tsp chopped garlic ✓ 1 tsp smoked paprika ✓ ½ tsp kosher salt ✓ 2 tsp fresh thyme leaves, roughly chopped ✓ 1½ pounds butternut squash, peeled, seeded, and cut into 1-inch cubes	✓ 1 large bunch chard, stems and leaves chopped ✓ 2 (15.5-oz) cans low-sodium chickpeas, drained and rinsed ✓ 32 ounces low-sodium chicken broth ✓ 1 tbsp freshly squeezed lemon juice ✓ 8 tsp grated Parmesan or Pecorino Romano cheese for garnish	❖ Place a soup pot, at least 4½ quarts in size, on the stove over medium heat. Add the chopped bacon and cook until the fat has rendered and the bacon is crisp. Remove the bacon pieces to a plate. ❖ Add the chopped onion and garlic to the same pot. Sauté in the bacon fat until the onion is soft, about 5 minutes. Add the paprika, salt, and thyme. Stir to coat the onion well. Add the squash, chard, chickpeas, and broth to the pot. ❖ Turn the heat to high, bring the soup to a boil, then turn the heat down to low and simmer until the squash is tender, about 20 minutes. ❖ Add the lemon juice. If necessary, add another pinch of salt to taste. ❖ Place 2 cups of cooled soup in each of 4 containers and top each serving with 2 tsp of cheese. Store the remaining 4 Servings: in the freezer to eat later. ❖ STORAGE: Store covered containers in the refrigerator for up to 5 days. If frozen, soup will last 4 months.

Nutrition: Total calories: 194; Total fat: 2g; Saturated fat: 1g; Sodium: 530mg; Carbohydrates: 34g; Fiber: 11g; Protein: 12g

100) TUNA SALAD ROLLS WITH HERBS

Cooking Time: 15 Minutes	Servings: 4

- ✓ 1 (11-ounce) pouch tuna in water
- ✓ 1 cup parsley leaves, chopped
- ✓ ¼ cup mint leaves, chopped
- ✓ ¼ cup minced shallot
- ✓ 1½ tsp sumac
- ✓ 1 tsp Dijon mustard
- ✓ 1 tbsp olive oil
- ✓ 1 tbsp freshly squeezed lemon juice

- ✓ ¼ cup unsalted sunflower seeds
- ✓ 16 large or medium romaine or bibb lettuce leaves
- ✓ 1 red bell pepper, cut into thin sticks (3 to 4 inches long)
- ✓ 3 Persian cucumbers, cut into thin sticks (3 to 4 inches long)

- ❖ In a large bowl, mix together the tuna, parsley, mint, shallot, sumac, mustard, oil, lemon juice, and sunflower seeds.
- ❖ Place ¾ cup of tuna salad in each of 4 containers. Place 4 lettuce leaves, one quarter of the peppers, and one quarter of the cucumbers in each of 4 separate containers so that they don't get soggy from the tuna salad.
- ❖ STORAGE: Store covered containers in the refrigerator for up to 4 days.
- ❖ TIP Tuna in pouches is preferable to cans, because pouches don't need to be drained and the tuna isn't soggy. You can substitute canned salmon, canned sardines, or even shredded rotisserie chicken for the tuna in this salad.

101) ITALIAN -STYLE POTATO SALAD

Cooking Time: 30 Minutes	Servings: 6

- ✓ 3 tbsp extra virgin olive oil
- ✓ ½ cup of sliced olives
- ✓ 1 tbsp olive juice
- ✓ 3 tbsp lemon juice, freshly squeezed is best

- ✓ 2 tbsp of mint, fresh and torn
- ✓ ¼ tsp sea salt
- ✓ 2 stalks of sliced celery
- ✓ 2 pounds baby potatoes
- ✓ 2 tbsp of chopped oregano, fresh is best

- ❖ Cut the potatoes into inch cubes.
- ❖ Toss the potatoes into a medium saucepan and cover them with water.
- ❖ Place the saucepan on the stove over high heat.
- ❖ Once the potatoes start to boil, bring the heat down to medium-low.
- ❖ Let the potatoes simmer for 13 to 1minutes. When you poke the potatoes with a fork and they feel tender, they are done.
- ❖ As the potatoes are simmering, grab a small bowl and mix the oil, olive juice, lemon juice, and salt. Whisk the ingredients together well.
- ❖ Once the potatoes are done, drain them and pour the potatoes into a bowl.
- ❖ Take the juice mixture and pour 3 tbsp over the potatoes right away.
- ❖ Combine the potatoes with the celery and olives.
- ❖ Prior to serving, sprinkle the potatoes with the mint, oregano, and rest of the dressing.

102) ITALIAN -STYLE ZUCCHINI NOODLES

Cooking Time: 10 Minutes	Servings: 2

- ✓ 2 large zucchini or 1 package of store-bought zucchini noodles
- ✓ 1 tsp olive oil
- ✓ 4 cloves garlic diced
- ✓ 10 oz cherry tomatoes cut in half
- ✓ 2-4 oz plain hummus
- ✓ 1 tsp oregano
- ✓ 1/2 tsp red wine vinegar plus more to taste

- ✓ 1/2 cup jarred artichoke hearts, drained and chopped
- ✓ 1/4 cup sun-dried tomatoes, drained and chopped
- ✓ Salt, to taste
- ✓ Pepper to taste
- ✓ Parmesan and fresh basil for topping

- ❖ Prepare the zucchini by cutting of the ends off zucchini and spiralize, set aside
- ❖ In a pan over medium heat, add in olive oil
- ❖ Then add in the garlic and cherry tomatoes to the pan, sauté until tomatoes begin to burst, about to 4 minutes
- ❖ Add in the zucchini noodles, sun-dried tomatoes, hummus, oregano, artichoke hearts and red wine vinegar to the pan, sauté for 1-2 minutes, or until zucchini is tender-crisp and heated through
- ❖ Season to taste with salt and pepper as needed
- ❖ Allow the zoodle to cool
- ❖ Distribute among the containers, store in the fridge for 2-3 days
- ❖ To Serve: Reheat in the microwave for 30 seconds or until heated through, serve immediately with parmesan and fresh basil. Enjoy

Nutrition: Calories:241;Carbs: 8g;Total Fat: 37g;Protein: 10g

103)   LOBSTER SALAD

	Cooking Time: 15 Minutes	Servings: 2

Ingredients:

- ¼ yellow onion, chopped
- ¼ yellow bell pepper, seeded and chopped
- ¾ pound cooked lobster meat, shredded
- ✓ 1 celery stalk, chopped
- ✓ Black pepper, to taste
- ✓ ¼ cup avocado mayonnaise

Directions:

- ❖ Mix together all the ingredients in a bowl and stir until well combined.
- ❖ Refrigerate for about 3 hours and serve chilled.
- ❖ Put the salad into a container for meal prepping and refrigerate for about 2 days.

Nutrition: Calories: 336 ;Carbohydrates: 2g;Protein: 27.2g;Fat: 25.2g ;Sugar: 1.2g;Sodium: 926mg

104)   CHICKEN WITH ITALIAN -STYLE PESTO

	Cooking Time: 40 Minutes	Servings: 4

Ingredients:

- ✓ 1 pound chicken breasts (2 large breasts), butterflied and cut in half to make 4 pieces
- ✓ 1 (6-ounce) jar prepared pesto
- ✓ 1 tsp olive oil
- ✓ 12 ounces baby spinach leaves
- ✓ Chunky Roasted Cherry Tomato and Basil Sauce

Directions:

- ❖ Place the chicken and pesto in a gallon-size resealable bag. Marinate for at least hour.
- ❖ Preheat the oven to 350°F and rub a 13-by-9-inch glass or ceramic baking dish with the oil, or spray with cooking spray.
- ❖ Place the spinach in the pan, then place the chicken on top of the spinach. Pour the pesto from the bag into the dish. Cover the pan with aluminum foil and bake for 20 minutes. Remove the foil and bake for another 15 to 20 minutes. Cool.
- ❖ Place 1 piece of chicken, one quarter of the spinach, and ⅓ cup of chunky tomato sauce in each of separate containers.
- ❖ STORAGE: Store covered containers in the refrigerator for up to days.

Nutrition: Total calories: 531; Total fat: 43g; Saturated fat: 7g; Sodium: 1,243mg; Carbohydrates: 13g; Fiber: 4g; Protein: 29g

105)   CRISPY BAKED CHICKEN

	Cooking Time: 40 Minutes	Servings: 2

Ingredients:

- ✓ 2 chicken breasts, skinless and boneless
- ✓ 2 tbsp butter
- ✓ ¼ tsp turmeric powder
- ✓ Salt and black pepper, to taste
- ✓ ¼ cup sour cream

Directions:

- ❖ Preheat the oven to 360 degrees F and grease a baking dish with butter.
- ❖ Season the chicken with turmeric powder, salt and black pepper in a bowl.
- ❖ Put the chicken on the baking dish and transfer it in the oven.
- ❖ Bake for about 10 minutes and dish out to serve topped with sour cream.
- ❖ Transfer the chicken in a bowl and set aside to cool for meal prepping. Divide it into 2 containers and cover the containers. Refrigerate for up to 2 days and reheat in microwave before serving.

Nutrition: Calories: 304 ;Carbohydrates: 1.4g;Protein: 21g;Fat: 21.6g ;Sugar: 0.1g;Sodium: 137mg

106) VEGETARIAN LASAGNA CANNELLONI

Cooking Time: 1 Hour 10 Minutes	**Servings: 14**

Ingredients:

- ✓ 1 pound lasagna noodles
- ✓ 3 thinly sliced zucchini, if your vegetables are smaller make it 4
- ✓ ½ cup water
- ✓ 3 tbsp olive oil
- ✓ Parmesan cheese and salt to taste
- ✓ 24-ounce jar of pasta sauce, you can use any type but the best for the recipes is basil or tomato
- ✓ Enough crushed red pepper flakes for your taste buds, this is also optional
- ✓ For the cheese filling:
- ✓ 6 ounces goat cheese
- ✓ 20 ounces of ricotta cheese
- ✓ 2 ounces mozzarella cheese
- ✓ 1 cup of parsley leaves, chopped
- ✓ Dash of salt and pepper
- ✓ 3 tbsp of chopped garlic
- ✓ Olive oil

Directions:

- ❖ Set the temperature of your oven to 450 degrees Fahrenheit.
- ❖ Grease a baking sheet or lay a piece of parchment paper on top.
- ❖ Slice the zucchini and place them on the baking sheet.
- ❖ Brush each side of the vegetable with oil and then sprinkle with salt.
- ❖ Place the baking sheet into the oven and set a timer for 10 minutes.
- ❖ While the zucchini is baking, start boiling the lasagna noodles. Drain the noodles when they are done cooking and then let them dry on a piece of parchment paper.
- ❖ Remove the zucchini from the oven and set aside to allow them to cool down a bit.
- ❖ Change the heat of your oven to 350 degrees Fahrenheit.
- ❖ To make the cheese filling, combine all of the ingredients and drizzle with a little olive oil. Mix well.
- ❖ Pour a spoonful or two on each of the lasagna noodles.
- ❖ Set a slice of baked zucchini on top of the cheese mixture.
- ❖ Roll up the noodles.
- ❖ In a 9 x inch baking pan, pour the water and ¾ cup of the pasta sauce on the bottom. Stir the ingredients gently so they become mixed.
- ❖ Place the lasagna roll-ups in the upright position on top of the sauce.
- ❖ Pour the remaining sauce on the noodles.
- ❖ If you want a little extra cheese, sprinkle some on top of the lasagna roll-ups.
- ❖ Set your timer for 40 minutes, but remember to check the liquid half-way through cooking to make sure it does not become too dry. If it does, add a little more water. You can try adding some water to the pasta sauce jar and shaking it up a bit as this will give the water a little sauce flavor.
- ❖ When the lasagna is cooked, remove it and garnish with basil leaves. Allow it to cool for a couple of minutes and admire your Italian -Style cooking skills before serving.

Nutrition: calories: 282, fats: 11 grams, carbohydrates: 29 grams, protein: 14.3 grams.

107) MILANESE CHICKEN

Cooking Time: 30 Minutes	**Servings: 6**

Ingredients:

- ✓ 4 skinless and boneless chicken breast halves
- ✓ 1 tbsp vegetable oil
- ✓ 2 garlic cloves, crushed
- ✓ 1 tsp Italian style seasoning
- ✓ 1 tsp crushed red pepper flakes
- ✓ salt
- ✓ pepper
- ✓ 1 28-ounce can stewed drained tomatoes
- ✓ 1 9-ounce package frozen green beans

Directions:

- ❖ Heat oil in a large skillet over medium-high heat.
- ❖ Add chicken to the skillet and season with garlic, red pepper, Italian seasoning, salt, and pepper.
- ❖ Saute for about 5 minutes.
- ❖ Add tomatoes and cook for 5 minutes more.
- ❖ Add green beans and give the whole mixture a gentle stir.
- ❖ Reduce heat, cover, and simmer for about 15-20 minutes.
- ❖ Enjoy!

Nutrition: Calories: 244, Total Fat: 4.9 g, Saturated Fat: 0.5 g, Cholesterol: mg, Sodium: 399 mg, Total Carbohydrate: 14.1 g, Dietary Fiber: 4.6 g, Total Sugars: 6.4 g, Protein: 38.2 g, Vitamin D: 0 mcg, Calcium: 48 mg, Iron: 3 mg, Potassium: 662 mg

108) CELERY TUNA SALAD

	Cooking Time: 30 Minutes	Servings: 4

✓ 3 5-ounce cans Genova tuna dipped in olive oil ✓ 2½ celery stalks, chopped ✓ ½ English cucumber, chopped ✓ 4-5 small radishes, stems removed, chopped ✓ 3 green onions, chopped (white and green) ✓ ½ medium red onion, finely chopped ✓ ½ cup pitted Kalamata olives, halved ✓ 1 bunch parsley, stems removed, finely chopped	✓ 10-15 sprigs fresh mint leaves, stems removed, finely chopped ✓ 6 slices heirloom tomatoes ✓ pita chips or pita bread ✓ 2½ tsp high-quality Dijon mustard ✓ zest of 1 lime ✓ lime juice, 1½ limes ✓ 1/3 cup olive oil ✓ ½ tsp sumac ✓ salt ✓ pepper ✓ ½ tsp crushed red pepper flakes	❖ Prepare the vinaigrette by combining and whisking all zesty Dijon mustard vinaigrette Ingredients: in a small bowl. ❖ For the tuna salad, add all base recipe Ingredients: to a large bowl, and mix well with a spoon. ❖ Dress the tuna salad with the prepared vinaigrette, and mix again until the tuna salad is coated correctly. ❖ Cover, refrigerate and allow to chill for 30 minutes. ❖ Once chilled, give the salad a toss and serve with a side of pita chips or pita bread and some sliced up heirloom tomatoes. ❖ Enjoy!

109) CHICKEN AND BUTTER WITH HERBS

	Cooking Time: 35 Minutes	Servings: 2

✓ 1/3 cup baby spinach ✓ 1 tbsp lemon juice ✓ ¾ pound chicken breasts ✓ 1/3 cup butter	✓ ¼ cup parsley, chopped ✓ Salt and black pepper, to taste ✓ 1/3 tsp ginger powder ✓ 1 garlic clove, minced	❖ Preheat the oven to 450 degrees F and grease a baking dish. ❖ Mix together parsley, ginger powder, lemon juice, butter, garlic, salt and black pepper in a bowl. ❖ Add chicken breasts in the mixture and marinate well for about minutes. ❖ Arrange the marinated chicken in the baking dish and transfer in the oven. ❖ Bake for about 2minutes and dish out to serve immediately. ❖ Place chicken in 2 containers and refrigerate for about 3 days for meal prepping. Reheat in microwave before serving.

110) ITALIAN-STYLE TUNA SANDWICHES

	Cooking Time: 10 Minutes	Servings: 4

✓ 3 tbsp lemon juice, freshly squeezed ✓ ½ tsp of minced garlic ✓ 5 ounces tuna, drained ✓ ½ cup of sliced olives	✓ 8 slices whole-grain bread ✓ 2 tbsp extra virgin olive oil ✓ ½ tsp black pepper ✓ 1 celery stalk, chopped	❖ Add the oil, pepper, lemon juice, and garlic to a bowl. Whisk the ingredients well. ❖ Combine the olives, chopped celery, and tuna. ❖ Use a fork to break apart the tuna into chunks. ❖ Stir all of the ingredients until they are well combined. ❖ Set four slices of bread on serving plates or a platter. ❖ Divide the tuna salad equally among the four slices of bread. ❖ Top the tuna salad with the remaining bread to make a sandwich. ❖ You'll get the best taste when you let the tuna sandwich sit for about 5 or more minutes before you serve. The salad will start to soak into the bread, and it makes for one tasty meal!

111)   BAKED FILLET OF SOLE ITALIAN STYLE

Cooking Time: 15 Minutes	Servings: 6

✓ 1 lime or lemon, juice of ✓ 1/2 cup extra virgin olive oil ✓ 3 tbsp unsalted melted vegan butter ✓ 2 shallots, thinly sliced ✓ 3 garlic cloves, thinly-sliced ✓ 2 tbsp capers ✓ 1.5 lb Sole fillet, about 10–12 thin fillets	✓ 4–6 green onions, top trimmed, halved lengthwise ✓ 1 lime or lemon, sliced (optional) ✓ 3/4 cup roughly chopped fresh dill for garnish ✓ 1 tsp seasoned salt, or to your taste ✓ 3/4 tsp ground black pepper ✓ 1 tsp ground cumin ✓ 1 tsp garlic powder	❖ Preheat over to 375-degree F ❖ In a small bowl, whisk together olive oil, lime juice, and melted butter with a sprinkle of seasoned salt, stir in the garlic, shallots, and capers. ❖ In a separate small bowl, mix together the pepper, cumin, seasoned salt, and garlic powder, season the fish fillets each on both sides. On a large baking pan or dish, arrange the fish fillets and cover with the buttery lime. Arrange the green onion halves and lime slices on top ❖ Bake in 375 degrees F for 10-15 minutes, do not overcook ❖ Remove the fish fillets from the oven. Allow the dish to cool completely Distribute among the containers, store for 2-3 days ❖ To Serve: Reheat in the microwave for 1-2 minutes or until heated through. Garnish with the chopped fresh dill. Serve with your favorite and a fresh salad ❖ Recipe Notes: If you can't get your hands on a sole fillet, cook this recipe with a different white fish. Just remember to change the baking time since it will be different.

112)   BAKED CHICKEN BREAST

Cooking Time: 50 Minutes	Servings: 2

✓ 2 skinless and boneless chicken breasts (about 8 ounces each) ✓ salt ✓ ground black pepper ✓ 1/4 cup olive oil	✓ 1/4 cup freshly squeezed lemon juice ✓ 1 garlic clove, minced ✓ 1/2 tsp dried oregano ✓ 1/4 tsp dried thyme	❖ Preheat oven to a temperature of 400 degrees F. ❖ Season the chicken breasts carefully with salt and pepper on all sides. ❖ Place the chicken in a bowl. ❖ Take another bowl and add olive oil, lemon juice, oregano, garlic, and thyme. Mix well to make the marinade. ❖ Pour the marinade on top of chicken breasts and allow to marinate for 10 minutes. ❖ Set an oven rack about inches above the heat source. ❖ Place the chicken breasts into a baking pan and pour extra marinade on top. Bake for about 35-45 minutes until the center is no longer pink and the juices run clear. ❖ Move the baking dish to top rack and broil for about 5 minutes. ❖ Cool, spread over containers with some side dish and enjoy!

113)   SALMON SKILLET LUNCH

Cooking Time: 15 To 20 Minutes	Servings: 4

✓ 1 tsp minced garlic ✓ 1 1/2 cup quartered cherry tomatoes ✓ 1 tbsp water ✓ 1/4 tsp sea salt ✓ 1 tbsp lemon juice, freshly squeezed is best	✓ 1 tbsp extra virgin olive oil ✓ 12 ounces drained and chopped roasted red peppers ✓ 1 tsp paprika ✓ 1/4 tsp black pepper ✓ 1 pound salmon fillets	❖ Remove the skin from your salmon fillets and cut them into 8 pieces. ❖ Turn your stove burner on medium heat and set a skillet on top. Pour the olive oil into the skillet and let it heat up for a couple of minutes. ❖ Add the minced garlic and paprika. Saute the ingredients for 1 minute. ❖ Combine the roasted peppers, black pepper, tomatoes, water, and salt. ❖ Set the heat to medium-high and bring the ingredients to a simmer. This should take 3 to 4 minutes. Remember to stir the ingredients occasionally so the tomatoes don't burn. Add the salmon and take some of the sauce from the skillet to spoon on top of the fish so it is all covered in the mixture. ❖ Cover the skillet and set a timer for 10 minutes. When the fish reaches 145 degrees Fahrenheit, it is cooked thoroughly. Turn off the heat and drizzle lemon juice over the fish. ❖ Break up the salmon into chunks and gently mix the pieces of fish with the sauce. Serve and enjoy!

Chapter 3

DINNER

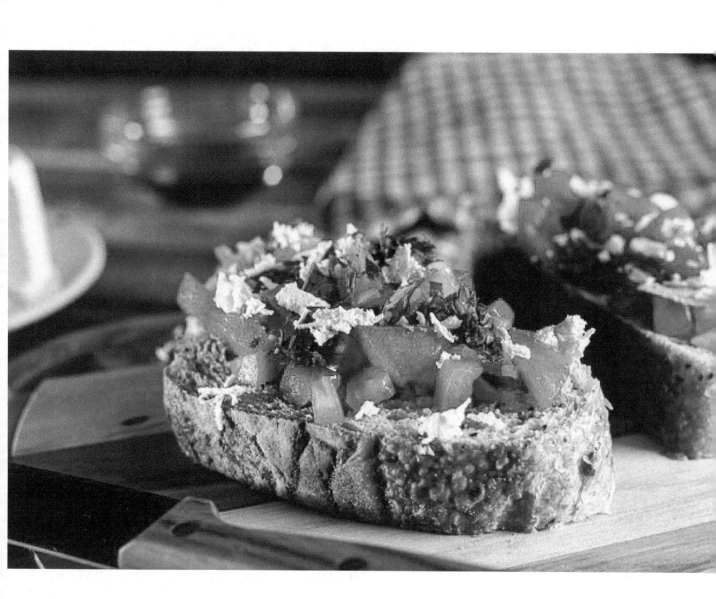

114) EASY ZUCCHINI SALAD WITH POMEGRANATE DRESSING

Preparation Time: 8 minutes	Cooking Time: 15 minutes	Servings: 6

Ingredients:

- ✓ One bunch of chives
- ✓ One pomegranate
- ✓ 1 tbsp pomegranate molasses
- ✓ 1/2 orange juice
- ✓ 1/4 cup mint leaf
- ✓ 120 g feta cheese
- ✓ 2 Lebanese cucumbers
- ✓ 2 tbsp currants
- ✓ 2 tbsp olive oil
- ✓ Three zucchinis
- ✓ salt and pepper

Directions:

- ❖ Clean the zucchini, then cucumber and slice the cucumber and cut it into ribbons using a peeler. And the same thing about your zucchini. Put the cucumber in the fridge.
- ❖ Chop chives into 2cm chunks and chop mint loosely.
- ❖ Make an orange Juice and combine with olive oil, a touch of pepper and salt, and 1 tbsp of pomegranate molasses to make the dressing. Whisk to blend.
- ❖ Toss the cucumber and zucchini into the dressing and apply the sliced herbs to prepare the salad.
- ❖ Add flowers and finish with the crumbled feta cheese.
- ❖ Slice the pomegranate into half and touch the skin's back with the dessert spoon to scatter the seeds over the salad.
- ❖ Now Serve.

Nutrition: Calories: 177.7 kcal Fat: 9.8 g Protein: 5.7 g Carbs: 20 g Fiber: 3.9 g

115) ITALIAN-STYLE GRAIN SALAD

Preparation Time: 5 minutes	Cooking Time: 35 minutes	Servings: 1

Ingredients:

- ✓ Coarse salt to taste
- ✓ Black pepper 2 tsp olive oil 1/2 minced small shallot 1/2 cup parsley, chopped 1
- ✓ 1 tbsp red wine vinegar 1 oz goat cheese, crumbled 1 cup grape tomatoes, halved

Directions:

- ❖ Combine the bulgur with 1/4 tsp salt and 1 cup of boiling water in a heat-proof dish. Cover, and let rest for about 30 minutes, before tender but somewhat chewy.
- ❖ Drain the bulgur and press to extract liquid in the fine-mesh sieve; return to the bowl. Add the onions, parsley, vinegar, shallot, and oil. Then season with pepper and salt, and toss.
- ❖ Top with cheese.

Nutrition: Calories:303 kcal Fat: 21g Protein: 10g Carbs: 21g Fiber: 4g

116) TROPICAL MACADAMIA NUTS DRESSING

Preparation Time: 10 minutes	Cooking Time: 10 minutes	Servings: 4

Ingredients:

- ✓ ¼ tsp onion powder
- ✓ ½ tsp pepper
- ✓ 1 cup Cashew Milk
- ✓ 1 cup Macadamia Nuts
- ✓ 1 tbsp chives, chopped
- ✓ 1 tbsp lemon juice
- ✓ 1 tsp apple cider vinegar
- ✓ 1 tsp garlic powder
- ✓ 1 tsp salt
- ✓ 2 tbsp parsley

Directions:

- ❖ A high-powered mixer and places all the ingredients (other than green onions and chives, and parsley). Start at low and bring it up to high speed steadily until the ingredients are fully blended. If you want a thinner consistency, add more Homemade Cashew Milk from Nature's Eats.
- ❖ Add now the diced chives and parsley, then blend until smooth.
- ❖ Now serve promptly or store it in the refrigerator in an air-tight bag.

Nutrition: Calories: 302 kcal Fat: 26 g Protein: 8 g Carbs: 19 g Fiber: 6.3 g

117) EASY VINAIGRETTE DRESSING

Preparation Time: 5 minutes	Cooking Time: 5 minutes	Servings: 1

- ✓ black pepper, to taste
- ✓ 3 tbsp vinegar
- ✓ Two cloves garlic, minced
- ✓ 1 tbsp honey
- ✓ 1 tbsp Dijon mustard
- ✓ ½ cup olive oil
- ✓ ¼ tsp salt

❖ Combine all the ingredients in a liquid mixing cup. With a small spoon or a fork, stir well till ingredients are thoroughly mixed together.

❖ Now taste, and customize as needed. Thin it out with a little more olive oil if the mixture becomes too acidic, or balance the flavors with a bit more maple, honey, or syrup. Add a pinch of salt if the mixture is a bit blah. If the zing is not enough, apply a tsp of vinegar.

❖ Serve instantly, or for potential use, cover, and refrigerate. For 7 to 10 days, the homemade vinaigrette lasts well. If the vinaigrette solidifies in the fridge somewhat, don't think about it. It helps to do this with real olive oil. Simply let it for 5 to 10 minutes at room temperature or microwave very quickly (approximately 20 secs) to liquefy that olive oil again. Now serve.

118) Greek style turkey burger with Tzatziki sauce

Preparation Time: 36 minutes	Cooking Time: 10 minutes	Servings: 4

- ✓ Turkey Burgers
- ✓ 1 lb ground turkey
- ✓ 1/3 cup chopped sun-dried tomatoes
- ✓ ½ cup chopped spinach leaves
- ✓ 1/4 cup chopped red onion
- ✓ 2 pressed garlic cloves
- ✓ ¼ cup feta cheese
- ✓ One egg
- ✓ 1 tsp dried oregano
- ✓ 1 tbsp olive oil
- ✓ 1/2 tsp kosher salt
- ✓ One sliced red onion
- ✓ Four hamburger buns
- ✓ 1/2 tsp ground black pepper
- ✓ A handful of Bibb lettuce leaves
- ✓ Tzatziki Sauce
- ✓ ½ grated cucumber
- ✓ Two minced garlic cloves
- ✓ 3/4 cup Greek yogurt
- ✓ 1 tbsp red wine vinegar
- ✓ One pinch of kosher salt
- ✓ 1 tbsp chopped dill
- ✓ One pinch of black pepper

❖ Combine all the ingredients of Tzatziki sauce in a bowl and mix well.

❖ Mix turkey, onion, sun-dried tomatoes, and feta cheese in a bowl.

❖ In another bowl, mix olive oil, egg, garlic, salt, oregano, and pepper.

❖ Pour egg mixture with turkey mixture. Mix well.

❖ Make medium-sized patties out of turkey mixture. Set aside in the refrigerator for 24 hours.

❖ Cook turkey patties on heated grill sprayed with oil for seven minutes from both sides on medium flame.

❖ Spread Tzatziki sauce over buns and place lettuce, onions, and cooked patties and serve.

119) SAUCY GREEK-STYLE BAKED SHRIMP

Preparation Time: 15 minutes	Cooking Time: 20 minutes	Servings: 4

- ✓ 2 tbsp chopped dill
- ✓ 1 lb shrimp
- ✓ 1/4 tsp kosher salt
- ✓ 1/2 tsp red pepper flakes
- ✓ 3 tbsp olive oil
- ✓ Three minced garlic cloves
- ✓ One chopped onion
- ✓ 15 oz crushed tomatoes
- ✓ 1/2 tsp ground cinnamon
- ✓ 1/2 tsp ground allspice
- ✓ 1/2 cup crumbled feta cheese

❖ Add salt, shrimps, and pepper in a bowl. Toss well and keep it aside.

❖ Cook garlic and onions in heated olive oil over medium flame for five minutes.

❖ Add spices and stir for half a minute.

❖ Mix tomatoes and let it simmer for 20 minutes with occasional stirring.

❖ Transfer the tomato mixture to the baking sheet and add shrimps to it. Spread cheese and bake in a preheated oven at 375 degrees for 20 minutes.

❖ Drizzle dill and serve.

Nutrition: Calories: 190 kcal Fat: 5.2 g Protein: 25.9 g Carbs: 11.9 g Fiber: 5.2 g

120) TASTY SAUTÉED CHICKEN WITH OLIVES CAPERS AND LEMONS

Preparation Time: 5 minutes	Cooking Time: 30 minutes	Servings: 4

Ingredients:

- ✓ Six boneless chicken thighs
- ✓ Two sliced lemons
- ✓ One minced garlic clove minced
- ✓ 2/4 cup extra virgin olive oil
- ✓ 2 tbsp all-purpose flour
- ✓ 2 tbsp butter
- ✓ 1 cup chicken broth
- ✓ kosher salt to taste
- ✓ 3/4 cup Sicilian green olives
- ✓ 2 tbsp parsley
- ✓ 1/4 cup capers
- ✓ Black pepper to taste

Directions:

- ❖ Add salt, chicken, and pepper in a bowl and toss well. Set aside for 15 minutes.
- ❖ Cook lemon slices (half of them) in heated olive oil over medium flame for five minutes from both sides.
- ❖ Shift the cooked brown lemon slices on the plate.
- ❖ Coat chicken pieces with rice flour and cook in heated olive oil in the skillet for seven minutes from both sides. Transfer the cooked chicken to the plate.
- ❖ Sauté garlic in heated oil in the same pan for about half a minute. Stir in olives, chicken broth, lemons, and capers. Cook over high flame for few minutes.
- ❖ When half of the broth is left, add parsley and butter. Cook for one minute.
- ❖ Add salt and pepper to adjust the taste and serve.

Nutrition: Calories: 595 kcal Fat: 34 g Protein: 51 g Carbs: 5.5 g Fiber: 9 g

121) ENGLISH PORRIDGE (OATMEAL)

Preparation Time: 2 minutes	Cooking Time: 2 minutes	Servings: 1

Ingredients:

- ✓ Base Recipe
- ✓ ½ cup oats
- ✓ 1/2cup water
- ✓ 1/2cup milk
- ✓ 1 Pinch salt
- ✓ Maple Brown Sugar
- ✓ 1 tsp sugar
- ✓ 2 tbsp chopped pecans
- ✓ 1 tsp maple syrup
- ✓ 1/8 tsp cinnamon
- ✓ Banana Nut
- ✓ ½ banana sliced
- ✓ 1 tbsp flaxseed
- ✓ 2 tbsp walnuts
- ✓ 1/8 tsp cinnamon
- ✓ Strawberry & Cream
- ✓ 1/2cup strawberries
- ✓ 2 tsp honey
- ✓ 1 tbsp half and half
- ✓ 1/8 tsp vanilla extract
- ✓ Chocolate Peanut Butter
- ✓ 2 tsp cocoa powder
- ✓ 2 tsp chocolate chips
- ✓ 1 tbsp peanut butter
- ✓ 1 tsp roasted peanuts

Directions:

- ❖ Microwave Instructions
- ❖ Place all the ingredients heat in the microwave on high for 2 minutes. Then add 15-sec increments until the oatmeal is puffed and softened.
- ❖ Stovetop Instructions
- ❖ Bring the water and milk to a boil in a pan. Lower the heat & pour in the oats. Cook it while stirring, till the oats are soft and have absorbed most of the liquid. Turn off the stove and let it for 2 to 3 min.
- ❖ Assembly
- ❖ Stir in the toppings and let rest for a few minutes to cool. Serve warm.

Nutrition: Calories: 227 kcal Fat:6 g Protein: 9 g Carbs: 33 g Fiber: 4 g

122) MOROCCAN SALAD FATTOUSH

Preparation Time: 20 minutes	Cooking Time: 20 minutes	Servings: 6

Ingredients:

- ✓ Two loaves of pita bread
- ✓ • ½ tsp sumac
- ✓ • Olive Oil
- ✓ • Salt and pepper
- ✓ • One chopped English cucumber
- ✓ • One chopped lettuce
- ✓ • Five chopped Roma tomatoes
- ✓ Five radishes
- ✓ • Five chopped green onions
- ✓ • 2 cup parsley leaves
- ✓ Lime-vinaigrette
- ✓ • 1/4 tsp cinnamon
- ✓ • 1 tsp lime juice
- ✓ • Salt and pepper
- ✓ • 1/3 cup Virgin Olive Oil
- ✓ • 1 tsp sumac
- ✓ • 1/4 tsp allspice

Directions:

- ❖ Toast the bread in the oven. Heat olive oil and fry until browned. Add salt, pepper, and 1/2tsp of sumac. Turn off heat & place pita chips on paper towels to drain.
- ❖ In a mixing bowl, mix the chopped lettuce, cucumber, tomatoes, green onions with the sliced radish and parsley.
- ❖ For seasoning, whisk the lemon or lime juice, olive oil, and spices in a small bowl.
- ❖ Sprinkle the salad & toss lightly. Finally, add the pita chips and more sumac if you like. Shifts to small serving bowls or plates. Enjoy!

Nutrition: Calories: 345 kcal Fat:20.4 g Protein: 9.1 g Carbs:39.8 g Fiber: 1 g

123) CALABRIA CICORIA E FAGIOLI

Preparation Time:	Cooking Time:	Servings: 6

Ingredients:

- ✓ 200 g dried cannellini beans
- ✓ • 6 tbsp olive oil
- ✓ • 400 g curly endive
- ✓ Four garlic cloves
- ✓ • 600 ml of water
- ✓ • Two red chilies
- ✓ • Salt and pepper to taste

Directions:

- ❖ Put the dried beans to soak for 12 h (they increase in size). Drain them and boil for two h in fresh unsalted water. Salt at the end of the cooking time. If using canned beans, drain them from their liquid and rinse them before use. Rinse the endive and cut it up into short lengths.
- ❖ Heat the olive oil, fry the garlic without browning, and then add the endive and chilies. Keeping the heat high, stir-fry for a minute or two, coating the endive with the oil, then add the drained cannellini beans, some salt, and the water. Bring to the boil, cover the pan, and lower the heat. Cook until the endive is soft and most of the liquid has been absorbed.

Nutrition: Calories:225 kcal Fat: 21 g Protein: 3 g Carbs: 6 g Fiber:1 g

124) CAMPANIA POACHED EGGS CAPRESE

Preparation Time: 10 minutes	Cooking Time: 10 minutes	Servings: 2

Ingredients:

- ✓ 4 tsp pesto
- ✓ • 1 tbsp white vinegar
- ✓ • Four eggs
- ✓ • 2 tsp salt
- ✓ 2 English muffins
- ✓ • salt to taste
- ✓ • One tomato sliced
- ✓ • Four slices of mozzarella cheese

Directions:

- ❖ Fill 2 to 3 inches of a pan with water and boil over a high flame. Lower the heat, add the vinegar, 2 tsp of salt in it, and let it simmer.
- ❖ Put a cheese slice and a slice of tomato on every English muffin half and put in a toaster oven for 5 min or till the cheese melts and the English muffin is well toasted.
- ❖ Break an egg in a bowl and add in the water one by one. Let the eggs cook for 2.5 to 3 minutes or until the yolks have solidified and the egg whites are firm. Take the eggs out of the water and put them on a kitchen towel to absorb excess water.
- ❖ For assembling, first put an egg on top of every muffin, add a tsp of pesto sauce on the egg, and scatter the salt.

125) GREEK BREAKFAST DISH WITH EGGS AND VEGETABLES

Preparation Time: 10 minutes	Cooking Time: 10 minutes	Servings: 2

Ingredients:

- ✓ 1 tbsp olive oil
- ✓ • salt to taste
- ✓ • 2 cup chopped rainbow chard
- ✓ • ½ cup arugula
- ✓ 1 cup spinach
- ✓ • Two cloves garlic
- ✓ • ½ cup grated Cheddar cheese
- ✓ • Four eggs
- ✓ • black pepper to taste

Directions:

- ❖ Heat oil over moderate pressure. Sauté the chard, spinach, and arugula until soft, around three minutes. Add garlic, continue cooking until aromatic, approx. Two min.
- ❖ In a cup, combine the eggs and the cheese; dump into the mixture of the chard. Heat and cook for 5 - 6 minutes. Season to taste with salt and pepper.

126) ITALIAN BREAKFAST PITA PIZZA

Preparation Time: 25 minutes	Cooking Time: 30 minutes	Servings: 2

Ingredients:

- ✓ Four slices of bacon
- ✓ 2 tbsp olive oil
- ✓ 1/4 onion
- ✓ Four eggs
- ✓ Two pita bread rounds
- ✓ 2 tbsp pesto
- ✓ ½ tomato
- ✓ One avocado
- ✓ ½ cup slashed spinach
- ✓ 1/4 cup mushrooms
- ✓ ½ cup grated Cheddar cheese

Directions:

- ❖ Heat the oven to 350 ° F (175° C).
- ❖ In a medium saucepan, put the bacon and cook over medium-high heat, rotating periodically, when browned uniformly, around ten minutes. Cook the onion in the same skillet till smooth. Put it aside. In the skillet, melt the olive oil. Add the eggs and cook, stirring regularly, for 3 to 5 minutes.
- ❖ Add the pita bread to the cake pan. Cover with bacon, fried eggs, onions, mushrooms, and spinach; sprinkle the pesto over through the pita. Dress over the toppings of Cheddar cheese.
- ❖ Bake it in the preheated oven for10 min. Serve with avocado pieces.

127) NAPOLI CAPRESE ON TOAST

Preparation Time: 15 minutes	Cooking Time: 5 minutes	Servings: 14

Ingredients:

- ✓ 14 slices bread
- ✓ 1 lb mozzarella cheese
- ✓ Two cloves garlic
- ✓ 1/3 cup basil leaves
- ✓ 3 tbsp olive oil
- ✓ Three tomatoes
- ✓ salt to taste
- ✓ black pepper to taste

Directions:

- ❖ Baked the bread slices and spread the garlic on one side of each piece. Put a slice of mozzarella cheese, 1 to 2 basil leaves, and a slice of tomato on each piece of toast. Sprinkle with olive oil, spray salt, and black pepper.

Nutrition: Calories: 203.5 kcal Fat: 10 g Protein: 10.5 g Carbs: 16.5 g Fiber: 1.1 g

128) TUSCAN EGGS FLORENTINE

Preparation Time: 10 minutes	Cooking Time: 10 minutes	Servings: 3

Ingredients:

- ✓ 2 tbsp butter
- ✓ Two cloves garlic
- ✓ 3 tbsp cream cheese
- ✓ ½ cup mushroom
- ✓ ½ fresh spinach
- ✓ Salt to taste
- ✓ Six eggs
- ✓ Black pepper to taste

Directions:

- ❖ Put the butter in a non-stick skillet; heat and mix the mushrooms and garlic till the garlic is flavorsome for about 1 min. Add spinach to the mushroom paste and cook until spinach is softened for 2 - 3 mins,
- ❖ Mix the mushroom-spinach mixer; add salt and pepper. Cook, with mixing, until the eggs are stiff; turn. Pour with cream cheese over the egg mixture and cook before cream cheese started melting just over five minutes.

Nutrition: Calories: 278.9 kcal Fat: 22.9 g Protein:15.7 g Carbs: 4.1 g Fiber:22.9

129) SPECIAL QUINOA, CEREALS FOR BREAKFAST

Preparation Time: 5 minutes	Cooking Time: 16 minutes	Servings: 4

Ingredients:

- ✓ 2 cups of water
- ✓ ½ cup apricots
- ✓ 1 cup quinoa
- ✓ ½ cup almonds
- ✓ 1 tsp cinnamon
- ✓ 1/3 cup seeds
- ✓ ½ tsp nutmeg

Directions:

- ❖ Combine water and quinoa in a medium saucepan and continue cooking. Lower the heat and boil when much of the water has been drained for 8–12 minutes. Whisk in apricots, almonds, linseeds, cinnamon, and nutmeg; simmer till the quinoa is soft.

Nutrition: Calories: 349.9 kcal Fat:15.1 g Protein: 11.8 g Carbs: 44.5 g Fiber: 9.3 g

130) SIMPLE ZUCCHINI WITH EGG

Preparation Time: 5 minutes	Cooking Time: 15 minutes	Servings: 2

Ingredients:

- ✓ Two eggs
- ✓ 1.5 tbsp olive oil
- ✓ salt to taste
- ✓ Two zucchinis
- ✓ Black pepper to taste
- ✓ 1 tsp water

Directions:

- ❖ Heat the oil in a saucepan over medium heat; sauté the zucchini until soft, around 10 minutes. Season with salt and black pepper.
- ❖ Add the eggs with a fork in a bowl; add more water and mix until uniformly mixed. Spill the eggs over the zucchini; continue cooking until the eggs are boiled and rubbery for almost 5 minutes. Dress it with salt and black pepper.

Nutrition: Calories: 21.7 kcal Fat: 15.7 g Protein: 10.2 g Carbs: 11.2 g Fiber: 3.6 g

131) ITALIAN BAKED EGGS IN AVOCADO

Preparation Time: 10 minutes	Cooking Time: 15 minutes	Servings: 2

- ✓ One pinch parsley
- ✓ Two eggs
- ✓ Two slice bacon
- ✓ One avocado
- ✓ 2 tsp chives
- ✓ One pinch of salt and black pepper

- ❖ Preheat the oven to 425 degrees.
- ❖ Break the eggs in a tub, willing to maintain the yolks preserved.
- ❖ Assemble the avocado halves in the baking bowl, rest them on the side. Slowly spoon one egg yolk in the avocado opening. Keep spooning the white egg into the hole till it is finished. Do the same with leftover egg yolk, egg white, and avocado. Dress with chives, parsley, sea salt, and pepper for each of the avocados.
- ❖ Gently put the baking dish in the preheated oven and cook for about 15 min well before the eggs are cooked. Sprinkle with bacon over the avocado.

132) SPECIAL GROUND PORK SKILLET

	Cooking Time: 25 Minutes	**Servings: 4**

✓ 1 ½ pounds ground pork ✓ 2 tbsp olive oil ✓ 1 bunch kale, trimmed and roughly chopped ✓ 1 cup onions, sliced ✓ 1/4 tsp black pepper, or more to taste	✓ 1/4 cup tomato puree ✓ 1 bell pepper, chopped ✓ 1 tsp sea salt ✓ 1 cup chicken bone broth ✓ 1/4 cup port wine ✓ 2 cloves garlic, pressed ✓ 1 chili pepper, sliced	❖ Heat tbsp of the olive oil in a cast-iron skillet over a moderately high heat. Now, sauté the onion, garlic, and peppers until they are tender and fragrant; reserve. ❖ Heat the remaining tbsp of olive oil; once hot, cook the ground pork and approximately 5 minutes until no longer pink. ❖ Add in the other ingredients and continue to cook for 15 to 17 minutes or until cooked through. ❖ Storing ❖ Place the ground pork mixture in airtight containers or Ziploc bags; keep in your refrigerator for up to 3 to 4 days. ❖ For freezing, place the ground pork mixture in airtight containers or heavy-duty freezer bags. Freeze up to 2 to 3 months. Defrost in the refrigerator. Bon appétit!

Nutrition: 349 Calories; 13g Fat; 4.4g Carbs; 45.3g Protein; 1.2g Fiber

133) DELICIOUS GREEK STYLE CHEESE PORK

	Cooking Time: 20 Minutes	**Servings: 6**

✓ 1 tbsp sesame oil ✓ 1 ½ pounds pork shoulder, cut into strips ✓ Himalayan salt and freshly ground black pepper, to taste ✓ 1/2 tsp cayenne pepper ✓ 1/2 cup shallots, roughly chopped	✓ 2 bell peppers, sliced ✓ 1/4 cup cream of onion soup ✓ 1/2 tsp Sriracha sauce ✓ 1 tbsp tahini (sesame butter ✓ 1 tbsp soy sauce ✓ 4 ounces gouda cheese, cut into small pieces	❖ Heat he sesame oil in a wok over a moderately high flame. ❖ Stir-fry the pork strips for 3 to 4 minutes or until just browned on all sides. Add in the spices, shallots and bell peppers and continue to cook for a further 4 minutes. ❖ Stir in the cream of onion soup, Sriracha, sesame butter, and soy sauce; continue to cook for to 4 minutes more. ❖ Top with the cheese and continue to cook until the cheese has melted. ❖ Storing ❖ Place your stir-fry in six airtight containers or Ziploc bags; keep in your refrigerator for 3 to 4 days. ❖ For freezing, wrap tightly with heavy-duty aluminum foil or freezer wrap. It will maintain the best quality for 2 to 3 months. Defrost in the refrigerator and reheat in your wok.

Nutrition: 424 Calories; 29.4g Fat; 3. Carbs; 34.2g Protein; 0.6g Fiber

134) SPECIAL PORK IN BLUE CHEESE SAUCE

	Cooking Time: 30 Minutes	**Servings: 6**

✓ 2 pounds pork center cut loin roast, boneless and cut into 6 pieces ✓ 1 tbsp coconut aminos ✓ 6 ounces blue cheese ✓ 1/3 cup heavy cream ✓ 1/3 cup port wine	✓ 1/3 cup roasted vegetable broth, preferably homemade ✓ 1 tsp dried hot chile flakes ✓ 1 tsp dried rosemary ✓ 1 tbsp lard ✓ 1 shallot, chopped ✓ 2 garlic cloves, chopped ✓ Salt and freshly cracked black peppercorns, to taste	❖ Rub each piece of the pork with salt, black peppercorns, and rosemary. ❖ Melt the lard in a saucepan over a moderately high flame. Sear the pork on all sides about 15 minutes; set aside. ❖ Cook the shallot and garlic until they've softened. Add in port wine to scrape up any brown bits from the bottom. ❖ Reduce the heat to medium-low and add in the remaining ingredients; continue to simmer until the sauce has thickened and reduced. ❖ Storing ❖ Divide the pork and sauce into six portions; place each portion in a separate airtight container or Ziploc bag; keep in your refrigerator for 3 to 4 days. ❖ Freeze the pork and sauce in airtight containers or heavy-duty freezer bags. Freeze up to 4 months. Defrost in the refrigerator. Bon appétit!

Nutrition: 34Calories; 18.9g Fat; 1.9g Carbs; 40.3g Protein; 0.3g Fiber

135) MISSISSIPPI-STYLE PULLED PORK

	Cooking Time: 6 Hours	Servings: 4

Ingredients	Ingredients	Directions
✓ 1 ½ pounds pork shoulder ✓ 1 tbsp liquid smoke sauce ✓ 1 tsp chipotle powder	✓ Au Jus gravy seasoning packet ✓ 2 onions, cut into wedges ✓ Kosher salt and freshly ground black pepper, taste	❖ Mix the liquid smoke sauce, chipotle powder, Au Jus gravy seasoning packet, salt and pepper. Rub the spice mixture into the pork on all sides. ❖ Wrap in plastic wrap and let it marinate in your refrigerator for 3 hours. ❖ Prepare your grill for indirect heat. Place the pork butt roast on the grate over a drip pan and top with onions; cover the grill and cook for about 6 hours. ❖ Transfer the pork to a cutting board. Now, shred the meat into bite-sized pieces using two forks. ❖ Storing ❖ Divide the pork between four airtight containers or Ziploc bags; keep in your refrigerator for up to 3 to 5 days. ❖ For freezing, place the pork in airtight containers or heavy-duty freezer bags. Freeze up to 4 months. Defrost in the refrigerator. Bon appétit!

136) SPICY WITH CHEESY TURKEY DIP

	Cooking Time: 25 Minutes	Servings: 4

Ingredients	Ingredients	Directions
✓ 1 Fresno chili pepper, deveined and minced ✓ 1 ½ cups Ricotta cheese, creamed, 4% fat, softened ✓ 1/4 cup sour cream ✓ 1 tbsp butter, room temperature ✓ 1 shallot, chopped	✓ 1 tsp garlic, pressed ✓ 1 pound ground turkey ✓ 1/2 cup goat cheese, shredded ✓ Salt and black pepper, to taste ✓ 1 ½ cups Gruyère, shredded	❖ Melt the butter in a frying pan over a moderately high flame. Now, sauté the onion and garlic until they have softened. ❖ Stir in the ground turkey and continue to cook until it is no longer pink. ❖ Transfer the sautéed mixture to a lightly greased baking dish. Add in Ricotta, sour cream, goat cheese, salt, pepper, and chili pepper. ❖ Top with the shredded Gruyère cheese. Bake in the preheated oven at 350 degrees F for about 20 minutes or until hot and bubbly in top. ❖ Storing ❖ Place your dip in an airtight container; keep in your refrigerator for up 3 to 4 days. Enjoy!

Nutrition: 284 Calories; 19g Fat; 3.2g Carbs; 26. Protein; 1.6g Fiber

137) TURKEY CHORIZO AND BOK CHOY

	Cooking Time: 50 Minutes	Servings: 4

Ingredients	Ingredients	Directions
✓ 4 mild turkey Chorizo, sliced ✓ 1/2 cup full-fat milk ✓ 6 ounces Gruyère cheese, preferably freshly grated ✓ 1 yellow onion, chopped	✓ Coarse salt and ground black pepper, to taste ✓ 1 pound Bok choy, tough stem ends trimmed ✓ 1 cup cream of mushroom soup ✓ 1 tbsp lard, room temperature	❖ Melt the lard in a nonstick skillet over a moderate flame; cook the Chorizo sausage for about 5 minutes, stirring occasionally to ensure even cooking; reserve. ❖ Add in the onion, salt, pepper, Bok choy, and cream of mushroom soup. Continue to cook for 4 minutes longer or until the vegetables have softened. ❖ Spoon the mixture into a lightly oiled casserole dish. Top with the reserved Chorizo. ❖ In a mixing bowl, thoroughly combine the milk and cheese. Pour the cheese mixture over the sausage. ❖ Cover with foil and bake at 36degrees F for about 35 minutes. ❖ Storing ❖ Cut your casserole into four portions. Place each portion in an airtight container; keep in your refrigerator for 3 to 4 days. ❖ For freezing, wrap your portions tightly with heavy-duty aluminum foil or freezer wrap. Freeze up to 1 to 2 months. Defrost in the refrigerator. Enjoy!

138) CLASSIC SPICY CHICKEN BREASTS

	Cooking Time: 30 Minutes	Servings: 6

Ingredients	Ingredients	Directions
✓ 1 ½ pounds chicken breasts ✓ 1 bell pepper, deveined and chopped ✓ 1 leek, chopped ✓ 1 tomato, pureed ✓ 2 tbsp coriander	✓ 2 garlic cloves, minced ✓ 1 tsp cayenne pepper ✓ 1 tsp dry thyme ✓ 1/4 cup coconut aminos ✓ Sea salt and ground black pepper, to taste	❖ Rub each chicken breasts with the garlic, cayenne pepper, thyme, salt and black pepper. Cook the chicken in a saucepan over medium-high heat. ❖ Sear for about 5 minutes until golden brown on all sides. ❖ Fold in the tomato puree and coconut aminos and bring it to a boil. Add in the pepper, leek, and coriander. ❖ Reduce the heat to simmer. Continue to cook, partially covered, for about 20 minutes. ❖ Storing ❖ Place the chicken breasts in airtight containers or Ziploc bags; keep in your refrigerator for 3 to 4 days. ❖ For freezing, place the chicken breasts in airtight containers or heavy-duty freezer bags. It will maintain the best quality for about 4 months. Defrost in the refrigerator. Bon appétit!

139) DELICIOUS SAUCY BOSTON BUTT

	Cooking Time: 1 Hour 20 Minutes	Servings: 8

Ingredients	Ingredients	Directions
✓ 1 tbsp lard, room temperature ✓ 2 pounds Boston butt, cubed ✓ Salt and freshly ground pepper ✓ 1/2 tsp mustard powder ✓ A bunch of spring onions, chopped	✓ 2 garlic cloves, minced ✓ 1/2 tbsp ground cardamom ✓ 2 tomatoes, pureed ✓ 1 bell pepper, deveined and chopped ✓ 1 jalapeno pepper, deveined and finely chopped ✓ 1/2 cup unsweetened coconut milk ✓ 2 cups chicken bone broth	❖ In a wok, melt the lard over moderate heat. Season the pork belly with salt, pepper and mustard powder. ❖ Sear the pork for 8 to 10 minutes, stirring periodically to ensure even cooking; set aside, keeping it warm. ❖ In the same wok, sauté the spring onions, garlic, and cardamom. Spoon the sautéed vegetables along with the reserved pork into the slow cooker. ❖ Add in the remaining ingredients, cover with the lid and cook for 1 hour 10 minutes over low heat. ❖ Divide the pork and vegetables between airtight containers or Ziploc bags; keep in your refrigerator for up to 3 to 5 days. ❖ For freezing, place the pork and vegetables in airtight containers or heavy-duty freezer bags. Freeze up to 4 months. Defrost in the refrigerator. Bon appétit!

140) SPECIAL OLD-FASHIONED HUNGARIAN GOULASH

	Cooking Time: 9 Hours 10 Minutes	Servings: 4

Ingredients	Ingredients	Directions
✓ 1 ½ pounds pork butt, chopped ✓ 1 tsp sweet Hungarian paprika ✓ 2 Hungarian hot peppers, deveined and minced ✓ 1 cup leeks, chopped ✓ 1 ½ tbsp lard ✓ 1 tsp caraway seeds, ground ✓ 4 cups vegetable broth ✓ 2 garlic cloves, crushed ✓ 1 tsp cayenne pepper ✓ 2 cups tomato sauce with herbs	✓ 1 ½ pounds pork butt, chopped ✓ 1 tsp sweet Hungarian paprika ✓ 2 Hungarian hot peppers, deveined and minced ✓ 1 cup leeks, chopped ✓ 1 ½ tbsp lard ✓ 1 tsp caraway seeds, ground ✓ 4 cups vegetable broth ✓ 2 garlic cloves, crushed ✓ 1 tsp cayenne pepper ✓ 2 cups tomato sauce with herbs	❖ Melt the lard in a heavy-bottomed pot over medium-high heat. Sear the pork for 5 to 6 minutes until just browned on all sides; set aside. ❖ Add in the leeks and garlic; continue to cook until they have softened. ❖ Place the reserved pork along with the sautéed mixture in your crock pot. Add in the other ingredients and stir to combine. ❖ Cover with the lid and slow cook for 9 hours on the lowest setting. ❖ Storing ❖ Spoon your goulash into four airtight containers or Ziploc bags; keep in your refrigerator for up to 3 to 4 days. ❖ For freezing, place the goulash in airtight containers. Freeze up to 4 to 6 months. Defrost in the refrigerator. Enjoy!

141) TYPICAL ITALIAN-STYLE CHEESY PORK LOIN

Cooking Time: 25 Minutes	**Servings: 4**

Ingredients:

- ✓ 1 pound pork loin, cut into 1-inch-thick pieces
- ✓ 1 tsp Italian seasoning mix
- ✓ Salt and pepper, to taste
- ✓ 1 onion, sliced
- ✓ 1 tsp fresh garlic, smashed
- ✓ 2 tbsp black olives, pitted and sliced
- ✓ 2 tbsp balsamic vinegar
- ✓ 1/2 cup Romano cheese, grated
- ✓ 2 tbsp butter, room temperature
- ✓ 1 tbsp curry paste
- ✓ 1 cup roasted vegetable broth
- ✓ 1 tbsp oyster sauce

Directions:

- ❖ In a frying pan, melt the butter over a moderately high heat. Once hot, cook the pork until browned on all sides; season with salt and black pepper and set aside.
- ❖ In the pan drippings, cook the onion and garlic for 4 to 5 minutes or until they've softened.
- ❖ Add in the Italian seasoning mix, curry paste, and vegetable broth. Continue to cook until the sauce has thickened and reduced slightly or about 10 minutes. Add in the remaining ingredients along with the reserved pork.
- ❖ Top with cheese and cook for 10 minutes longer or until cooked through.
- ❖ Storing
- ❖ Divide the pork loin between four airtight containers; keep in your refrigerator for 3 to 5 days.
- ❖ For freezing, place the pork loin in airtight containers or heavy-duty freezer bags. Freeze up to 4 to 6 months. Defrost in the refrigerator. Enjoy!

142) BAKED SPARE RIBS

Cooking Time: 3 Hour 40 Minutes	**Servings: 6**

Ingredients:

- ✓ 2 pounds spare ribs
- ✓ 1 garlic clove, minced
- ✓ 1 tsp dried marjoram
- ✓ 1 lime, halved
- ✓ Salt and ground black pepper, to taste

Directions:

- ❖ Toss all ingredients in a ceramic dish.
- ❖ Cover and let it refrigerate for 5 to 6 hours.
- ❖ Roast the foil-wrapped ribs in the preheated oven at 275 degrees F degrees for about hours 30 minutes.
- ❖ Storing
- ❖ Divide the ribs into six portions. Place each portion of ribs in an airtight container; keep in your refrigerator for 3 to days.
- ❖ For freezing, place the ribs in airtight containers or heavy-duty freezer bags. Freeze up to 4 to months. Defrost in the refrigerator and reheat in the preheated oven. Bon appétit!

143) HEALTHY CHICKEN PARMESAN SALAD

Cooking Time: 20 Minutes	**Servings: 6**

- ✓ 2 romaine hearts, leaves separated
- ✓ Flaky sea salt and ground black pepper, to taste
- ✓ 1/4 tsp chili pepper flakes
- ✓ 1 tsp dried basil
- ✓ 1/4 cup Parmesan, finely grated
- ✓ 2 chicken breasts
- ✓ 2 Lebanese cucumbers, sliced
- ✓ For the dressing:
- ✓ 2 large egg yolks
- ✓ 1 tsp Dijon mustard
- ✓ 1 tbsp fresh lemon juice
- ✓ 1/4 cup olive oil
- ✓ 2 garlic cloves, minced

Directions:

- ❖ In a grilling pan, cook the chicken breast until no longer pink or until a meat thermometer registers 5 degrees F. Slice the chicken into strips.
- ❖ Storing
- ❖ Place the chicken breasts in airtight containers or Ziploc bags; keep in your refrigerator for to 4 days.
- ❖ For freezing, place the chicken breasts in airtight containers or heavy-duty freezer bags. It will maintain the best quality for about months. Defrost in the refrigerator.
- ❖ Toss the chicken with the other ingredients. Prepare the dressing by whisking all the ingredients.
- ❖ Dress the salad and enjoy! Keep the salad in your refrigerator for 3 to 5 days.

144) CLASSIC TURKEY WINGS WITH GRAVY SAUCE

Cooking Time: 6 Hours	Servings: 6

Ingredients:

- ✓ 2 pounds turkey wings
- ✓ 1/2 tsp cayenne pepper
- ✓ 4 garlic cloves, sliced
- ✓ 1 large onion, chopped
- ✓ Salt and pepper, to taste
- ✓ 1 tsp dried marjoram
- ✓ 1 tbsp butter, room temperature
- ✓ 1 tbsp Dijon mustard
- ✓ For the Gravy:
- ✓ 1 cup double cream
- ✓ Salt and black pepper, to taste
- ✓ 1/2 stick butter
- ✓ 3/4 tsp guar gum

Directions:

- ❖ Rub the turkey wings with the Dijon mustard and tbsp of butter. Preheat a grill pan over medium-high heat.
- ❖ Sear the turkey wings for 10 minutes on all sides.
- ❖ Transfer the turkey to your Crock pot; add in the garlic, onion, salt, pepper, marjoram, and cayenne pepper. Cover and cook on low setting for 6 hours.
- ❖ Melt 1/2 stick of the butter in a frying pan. Add in the cream and whisk until cooked through.
- ❖ Next, stir in the guar gum, salt, and black pepper along with cooking juices. Let it cook until the sauce has reduced by half.
- ❖ Storing
- ❖ Wrap the turkey wings in foil before packing them into airtight containers; keep in your refrigerator for up to 3 to 4 days.
- ❖ For freezing, place the turkey wings in airtight containers or heavy-duty freezer bags. Freeze up to 2 to 3 months. Defrost in the refrigerator.
- ❖ Keep your gravy in refrigerator for up to 2 days.

145) AUTHENTIC PORK CHOPS WITH HERBS

Cooking Time: 20 Minutes	Servings: 4

Ingredients:

- ✓ 1 tbsp butter
- ✓ 1 pound pork chops
- ✓ 2 rosemary sprigs, minced
- ✓ 1 tsp dried marjoram
- ✓ 1 tsp dried parsley
- ✓ A bunch of spring onions, roughly chopped
- ✓ 1 thyme sprig, minced
- ✓ 1/2 tsp granulated garlic
- ✓ 1/2 tsp paprika, crushed
- ✓ Coarse salt and ground black pepper, to taste

- ❖ Season the pork chops with the granulated garlic, paprika, salt, and black pepper.
- ❖ Melt the butter in a frying pan over a moderate flame. Cook the pork chops for 6 to 8 minutes, turning them occasionally to ensure even cooking.
- ❖ Add in the remaining ingredients and cook an additional 4 minutes.
- ❖ Storing
- ❖ Divide the pork chops into four portions; place each portion in a separate airtight container or Ziploc bag; keep in your refrigerator for 3 to 4 days.
- ❖ Freeze the pork chops in airtight containers or heavy-duty freezer bags. Freeze up to 4 months. Defrost in the refrigerator. Bon appétit!

146) PEPPERS STUFFED WITH CHOPPED PORK ORIGINAL

Cooking Time: 40 Minutes	Servings: 4

Ingredients:

- ✓ 6 bell peppers, deveined
- ✓ 1 tbsp vegetable oil
- ✓ 1 shallot, chopped
- ✓ 1 garlic clove, minced
- ✓ 1/2 pound ground pork
- ✓ 1/3 pound ground veal
- ✓ 1 ripe tomato, chopped
- ✓ 1/2 tsp mustard seeds
- ✓ Sea salt and ground black pepper, to taste

- ❖ Parboil the peppers for 5 minutes.
- ❖ Heat the vegetable oil in a frying pan that is preheated over a moderate heat. Cook the shallot and garlic for 3 to 4 minutes until they've softened.
- ❖ Stir in the ground meat and cook, breaking apart with a fork, for about 6 minutes. Add the chopped tomatoes, mustard seeds, salt, and pepper.
- ❖ Continue to cook for 5 minutes or until heated through. Divide the filling between the peppers and transfer them to a baking pan.
- ❖ Bake in the preheated oven at 36degrees F approximately 25 minutes.
- ❖ Storing
- ❖ Place the peppers in airtight containers or Ziploc bags; keep in your refrigerator for up to 3 to 4 days.
- ❖ For freezing, place the peppers in airtight containers or heavy-duty freezer bags. Freeze up to 2 to 3 months. Defrost in the refrigerator. Bon appétit!

Nutrition: 2 Calories; 20.5g Fat; 8.2g Carbs; 18.2g Protein; 1.5g Fiber

147) GRILL-STYLE CHICKEN SALAD WITH AVOCADO

	Cooking Time: 20 Minutes	Servings: 4

Ingredients:

- 1/3 cup olive oil
- 2 chicken breasts
- Sea salt and crushed red pepper flakes
- 2 egg yolks
- ✓ 1 tbsp fresh lemon juice
- ✓ 1/2 tsp celery seeds
- ✓ 1 tbsp coconut aminos
- ✓ 1 large-sized avocado, pitted and sliced

Directions:

- ❖ Grill the chicken breasts for about 4 minutes per side. Season with salt and pepper, to taste.
- ❖ Slice the grilled chicken into bite-sized strips.
- ❖ To make the dressing, whisk the egg yolks, lemon juice, celery seeds, olive oil and coconut aminos in a measuring cup.
- ❖ Storing
- ❖ Place the chicken breasts in airtight containers or Ziploc bags; keep in your refrigerator for 3 to 4 days.
- ❖ For freezing, place the chicken breasts in airtight containers or heavy-duty freezer bags. It will maintain the best quality for about 4 months. Defrost in the refrigerator.
- ❖ Store dressing in your refrigerator for 3 to 4 days. Dress the salad and garnish with fresh avocado. Bon appétit!

148) EASY TO COOK RIBS

	Cooking Time: 8 Hours	Servings: 4

- 1 pound baby back ribs
- 4 tbsp coconut aminos
- 1/4 cup dry red wine
- 1/2 tsp cayenne pepper
- 1 garlic clove, crushed
- ✓ 1 tsp Italian herb mix
- ✓ 1 tbsp butter
- ✓ 1 tsp Serrano pepper, minced
- ✓ 1 Italian pepper, thinly sliced
- ✓ 1 tsp grated lemon zest

- ❖ Butter the sides and bottom of your Crock pot. Place the pork and peppers on the bottom.
- ❖ Add in the remaining ingredients.
- ❖ Slow cook for 9 hours on Low heat setting.
- ❖ Storing
- ❖ Divide the baby back ribs into four portions. Place each portion of the ribs along with the peppers in an airtight container; keep in your refrigerator for 3 to days.
- ❖ For freezing, place the ribs in airtight containers or heavy-duty freezer bags. Freeze up to 4 to months. Defrost in the refrigerator. Reheat in your oven at 250 degrees F until heated through.

149) CLASSIC BRIE-STUFFED MEATBALLS

	Cooking Time: 25 Minutes	Servings: 5

- 2 eggs, beaten
- 1 pound ground pork
- 1/3 cup double cream
- 1 tbsp fresh parsley
- Kosher salt and ground black pepper
- ✓ 1 tsp dried rosemary
- ✓ 10 (1-inch cubes of brie cheese
- ✓ 2 tbsp scallions, minced
- ✓ 2 cloves garlic, minced

- ❖ Mix all ingredients, except for the brie cheese, until everything is well incorporated.
- ❖ Roll the mixture into 10 patties; place a piece of cheese in the center of each patty and roll into a ball.
- ❖ Roast in the preheated oven at 0 degrees F for about 20 minutes.
- ❖ Storing
- ❖ Place the meatballs in airtight containers or Ziploc bags; keep in your refrigerator for up to 3 to 4 days.
- ❖ Freeze the meatballs in airtight containers or heavy-duty freezer bags. Freeze up to 3 to 4 months. To defrost, slowly reheat in a saucepan. Bon appétit!

Nutrition: 302 Calories; 13g Fat; 1.9g Carbs; 33.4g Protein; 0.3g Fiber

150) ITALIAN-STYLE CHICKEN WITH SWEET POTATO AND BROCCOLI

	Cooking Time: 30 Minutes	Servings: 8

Ingredients:

- ✓ 2 lbs boneless skinless chicken breasts, cut into small pieces
- ✓ 5-6 cups broccoli florets
- ✓ 3 tbsp Italian seasoning mix of your choice
- ✓ a few tbsp of olive oil
- ✓ 3 sweet potatoes, peeled and diced
- ✓ Coarse sea salt, to taste
- ✓ Freshly cracked pepper, to taste
- ✓ Toppings:
- ✓ Avocado
- ✓ Lemon juice
- ✓ Chives
- ✓ Olive oil, for serving

Directions:

- ❖ Preheat the oven to 425 degrees F
- ❖ Toss the chicken pieces with the Italian seasoning mix and a drizzle of olive oil, stir to combine then store in the fridge for about 30 minutes
- ❖ Arrange the broccoli florets and sweet potatoes on a sheet pan, drizzle with the olive oil, sprinkle generously with salt
- ❖ Arrange the chicken on a separate sheet pan
- ❖ Bake both in the oven for 12-1minutes
- ❖ Transfer the chicken and broccoli to a plate, toss the sweet potatoes and continue to roast for another 15 minutes, or until ready
- ❖ Allow the chicken, broccoli, and sweet potatoes to cool
- ❖ Distribute among the containers and store for 2-3 days
- ❖ To Serve: Reheat in the microwave for 1 minute or until heated through, top with the topping of choice. Enjoy
- ❖ Recipe Notes: Any kind of vegetables work will with this recipe! So, add favorites like carrots, brussels sprouts and asparagus.

Nutrition: Calories:222;Total Fat: 4.9g;Total Carbs: 15.3g;Protein: 28g

151) VEGETABLE SOUP

	Cooking Time: 20 Minutes	Servings: 6

Ingredients:

- ✓ 1 15-ounce can low sodium cannellini beans, drained and rinsed
- ✓ 1 tbsp olive oil
- ✓ 1 small onion, diced
- ✓ 2 carrots, diced
- ✓ 2 stalks celery, diced
- ✓ 1 small zucchini, diced
- ✓ 1 garlic clove, minced
- ✓ 1 tbsp fresh thyme leaves, chopped
- ✓ 2 tsp fresh sage, chopped
- ✓ ½ tsp salt
- ✓ ¼ tsp freshly ground black pepper
- ✓ 32 ounces low sodium chicken broth
- ✓ 1 14-ounce can no-salt diced tomatoes, undrained
- ✓ 2 cups baby spinach leaves, chopped
- ✓ 1/3 cup freshly grated parmesan

Directions:

- ❖ Mash half of the beans in a small bowl using the back of a spoon and put it to the side.
- ❖ Add the oil to a large soup pot and place over medium-high heat.
- ❖ Add carrots, onion, celery, garlic, zucchini, thyme, salt, pepper, and sage.
- ❖ Cook well for about 5 minutes until the vegetables are tender.
- ❖ Add broth and tomatoes and bring the mixture to a boil.
- ❖ Add beans (both mashed and whole) and spinach.
- ❖ Cook for 3 minutes until the spinach has wilted.
- ❖ Pour the soup into the jars.
- ❖ Before serving, top with parmesan.
- ❖ Enjoy!

Nutrition: Calories: 359, Total Fat: 7.1 g, Saturated Fat: 2.7 g, Cholesterol: 10 mg, Sodium: 854 mg, Total Carbohydrate: 51.1 g, Dietary Fiber: 20 g, Total Sugars: 5.7 g, Protein: 25.8 g, Vitamin D: 0 mcg, Calcium: 277 mg, Iron: 7 mg, Potassium: 1497 mg

152) GREEK-STYLE CHICKEN WRAPS

	Cooking Time: 15 Minutes	Servings: 2

✓ Greek Chicken Wrap Filling: ✓ 2 chicken breasts 14 oz, chopped into 1-inch pieces ✓ 2 small zucchinis, cut into 1-inch pieces ✓ 2 bell peppers, cut into 1-inch pieces ✓ 1 red onion, cut into 1-inch pieces ✓ 2 tbsp olive oil	✓ 2 tsp oregano ✓ 2 tsp basil ✓ 1/2 tsp garlic powder ✓ 1/2 tsp onion powder ✓ 1/2 tsp salt ✓ 2 lemons, sliced ✓ To Serve: ✓ 1/4 cup feta cheese crumbled ✓ 4 large flour tortillas or wraps	❖ Pre-heat oven to 425 degrees F ❖ In a bowl, toss together the chicken, zucchinis, olive oil, oregano, basil, garlic, bell peppers, onion powder, onion powder and salt ❖ Arrange lemon slice on the baking sheet(s), spread the chicken and vegetable out on top (use 2 baking sheets if needed) ❖ Bake for 15 minutes, until veggies are soft and the chicken is cooked through Allow to cool completely ❖ Distribute the chicken, bell pepper, zucchini and onions among the containers and remove the lemon slices Allow the dish to cool completely ❖ Distribute among the containers, store for 3 days ❖ To Serve: Reheat in the microwave for 1-2 minutes or until heated through. Wrap in a tortila and sprinkle with feta cheese. Enjoy

153) GARBANZO BEAN SOUP

	Cooking Time: 20 Minutes	Servings: 4

✓ 14 ounces diced tomatoes ✓ 1 tsp olive oil ✓ 1 15-ounce can garbanzo beans	✓ salt ✓ pepper ✓ 2 sprigs fresh rosemary ✓ 1 cup acini di pepe pasta	❖ Take a large saucepan and add tomatoes and ounces of the beans. ❖ Bring the mixture to a boil over medium-high heat. ❖ Puree the remaining beans in a blender/food processor. ❖ Stir the pureed mixture into the pan. ❖ Add the sprigs of rosemary to the pan. ❖ Add acini de Pepe pasta and simmer until the pasta is soft, making sure to stir it from time to time. ❖ Remove the rosemary. ❖ Season with pepper and salt. ❖ Enjoy!

154) ITALIAN SALAD OF SPINACH AND BEANS

	Cooking Time: 30 Minutes	Servings: 4

✓ 15 ounces drained and rinsed cannellini beans ✓ 14 ounces drained, rinsed, and quartered artichoke hearts ✓ 6 ounces or 8 cups baby spinach ✓ 14 ½ ounces undrained diced tomatoes, no salt is best ✓ 1 tbsp olive oil and any additional if you prefer	✓ ¼ tsp salt ✓ 2 minced garlic cloves ✓ 1 chopped onion, small in size ✓ ¼ tsp pepper ✓ ⅛ tsp crushed red pepper flakes ✓ 2 tbsp Worcestershire sauce	❖ Place a saucepan on your stovetop and turn the temperature to medium-high. ❖ Let the pan warm up for a minute before you pour in the tbsp of oil. Continue to let the oil heat up for another minute or two. ❖ Toss in your chopped onion and stir so all the pieces are bathed in oil. Saute the onions for minutes. ❖ Add the garlic to the saucepan. Stir and saute the ingredients for another minute. ❖ Combine the salt, red pepper flakes, pepper, and Worcestershire sauce. Mix well and then add the tomatoes to the pan. Stir the mixture constantly for about minutes. ❖ Add the artichoke hearts, spinach, and beans. Saute and stir occasionally to get the taste throughout the dish. Once the spinach starts to wilt, take the salad off of the heat. ❖ Serve and enjoy immediately to get the best taste.

Nutrition: calories: 1, fats: 4 grams, carbohydrates: 30 grams, protein: 8 grams.

155) SALMON SKILLET LUNCH

Cooking Time: 15 To 20 Minutes	Servings: 4

Ingredients	Ingredients	Instructions
✓ 1 tsp minced garlic ✓ 1 ½ cup quartered cherry tomatoes ✓ 1 tbsp water ✓ ¼ tsp sea salt ✓ 1 tbsp lemon juice, freshly squeezed is best	✓ 1 tbsp extra virgin olive oil ✓ 12 ounces drained and chopped roasted red peppers ✓ 1 tsp paprika ✓ ¼ tsp black pepper ✓ 1 pound salmon fillets	❖ Remove the skin from your salmon fillets and cut them into 8 pieces. ❖ Turn your stove burner on medium heat and set a skillet on top. Pour the olive oil into the skillet and let it heat up for a couple of minutes. ❖ Add the minced garlic and paprika. Saute the ingredients for 1 minute. ❖ Combine the roasted peppers, black pepper, tomatoes, water, and salt. ❖ Set the heat to medium-high and bring the ingredients to a simmer. This should take 3 to 4 minutes. Remember to stir the ingredients occasionally so the tomatoes don't burn. Add the salmon and take some of the sauce from the skillet to spoon on top of the fish so it is all covered in the mixture. ❖ Cover the skillet and set a timer for 10 minutes. When the fish reaches 145 degrees Fahrenheit, it is cooked thoroughly. Turn off the heat and drizzle lemon juice over the fish. ❖ Break up the salmon into chunks and gently mix the pieces of fish with the sauce. Serve and enjoy!

156) HALIBUT IN HERB CRUST

Cooking Time: 25 Minutes	Servings: 4

Ingredients	Ingredients	Instructions
✓ Fresh parsley (.33 cup) ✓ Fresh dill (.25 cup) ✓ Fresh chives (.25 cup) ✓ Lemon zest (1 tsp.) ✓ Panko breadcrumbs (.75 cup)	✓ Olive oil (1 tbsp.) ✓ Freshly cracked black pepper (.25 tsp.) ✓ Sea salt (1 tsp.) ✓ Halibut fillets (4 - 6 oz.)	❖ Chop the fresh dill, chives, and parsley. Prepare a baking tray using a sheet of foil. Set the oven to reach 400° Fahrenheit. ❖ Combine the salt, pepper, lemon zest, olive oil, chives, dill, parsley, and the breadcrumbs in a mixing bowl. ❖ Rinse the halibut thoroughly. Use paper towels to dry it before baking. ❖ Arrange the fish on the baking sheet. Spoon the crumbs over the fish and press it into each of the fillets. ❖ Bake it until the top is browned and easily flaked or about 10 to 1minutes.

157) SYRIAN SPICED BARLEY, LENTIL, AND VEGETABLE SOUP

Cooking Time: 40 Minutes	Servings: 5

Ingredients	Ingredients	Instructions
✓ 1 tbsp olive oil ✓ 1 small onion, chopped (about 2 cups) ✓ 2 medium carrots, peeled and chopped (about 1 cup) ✓ 1 celery stalk, chopped (about ½ cup) ✓ 1 tsp chopped garlic ✓ 1 tsp ground cumin ✓ 1 tsp ground coriander	✓ 1 tsp turmeric ✓ ⅛ tsp ground cinnamon ✓ 2 tbsp tomato paste ✓ ¾ cup green lentils ✓ ¾ cup pearled barley ✓ 8 cups water ✓ ¾ tsp kosher salt ✓ 1 (5-ounce) package baby spinach leaves ✓ 2 tsp red wine vinegar	❖ Heat the oil in a soup pot on medium-high heat. When the oil is shimmering, add the onion, carrots, celery, and garlic and sauté for 8 minutes. Add the cumin, coriander, turmeric, cinnamon, and tomato paste and cook for 2 more minutes, stirring frequently. ❖ Add the lentils, barley, water, and salt to the pot and bring to a boil. Turn the heat to low and simmer for minutes. Add the spinach and continue to simmer for 5 more minutes. ❖ Add the vinegar and adjust the seasoning if needed. ❖ Spoon 2 cups of soup into each of 5 containers. ❖ STORAGE: Store covered containers in the refrigerator for up to days.

Nutrition: Total calories: 273; Total fat: 4g; Saturated fat: 1g; Sodium: 459mg; Carbohydrates: 50g; Fiber: 1; Protein: 12g

158) CHICKEN WITH SPINACH

	Cooking Time: 20 Minutes	Servings: 2

Ingredients:

- ✓ 2 garlic cloves, minced
- ✓ 2 tbsp unsalted butter, divided
- ✓ ¼ cup parmesan cheese, shredded
- ✓ ¾ pound chicken tenders
- ✓ ¼ cup heavy cream
- ✓ 10 ounce frozen spinach, chopped
- ✓ Salt and black pepper, to taste

Directions:

- ❖ Heat tbsp of butter in a large skillet and add chicken, salt and black pepper.
- ❖ Cook for about 3 minutes on both sides and remove the chicken in a bowl.
- ❖ Melt remaining butter in the skillet and add garlic, cheese, heavy cream and spinach.
- ❖ Cook for about 2 minutes and transfer the chicken in it.
- ❖ Cook for about minutes on low heat and dish out to immediately serve.
- ❖ Place chicken in a dish and set aside to cool for meal prepping. Divide it in 2 containers and cover them. Refrigerate for about 3 days and reheat in microwave before serving.

Nutrition: Calories: 288 ;Carbohydrates: 3.6g;Protein: 27g;Fat: 18.3g;Sugar: 0.3g;Sodium: 192mg

159) SPINACH SALAD AND BLOOD ORANGE VINAIGRETTE

	Cooking Time: 10 Minutes	Servings: 6

Ingredients:

- ✓ ½ cup fresh blood orange juice
- ✓ 1/3 cup extra-virgin olive oil
- ✓ 2 tbsp sherry reserve vinegar
- ✓ 1 tbsp fresh grated ginger
- ✓ 1 tsp garlic powder
- ✓ 1 tsp ground sumac
- ✓ salt
- ✓ pepper
- ✓ 1/3 cup dried apricots, chopped
- ✓ 2 tbsp sherry reserve vinegar
- ✓ 2 loaves pita bread
- ✓ 2/3 cup vegetable oil
- ✓ 1/3 cup raw unsalted almonds
- ✓ 1/3 cup raw sliced almonds
- ✓ ½ tsp sumac
- ✓ ½ tsp paprika
- ✓ salt
- ✓ 4 cups baby spinach
- ✓ 3 cups frisee lettuce, chopped
- ✓ 2 shallots, thinly sliced
- ✓ 1-2 blood oranges, peeled and sliced crosswise

Directions:

- ❖ In a small bowl, soak the dried apricots in the sherry-reserved vinegar for about 5 minutes.
- ❖ Drain apricots and set aside.
- ❖ Toast pita bread until crispy and break into pieces.
- ❖ Heat vegetable oil in a frying pan over medium-high heat.
- ❖ Add broken pitas and almonds and fry them for a while.
- ❖ Add sliced up almonds, sumac, and paprika, and toss everything well.
- ❖ Remove from heat once the almonds show a golden brown color.
- ❖ Place on paper towels and allow to drain.
- ❖ In a mixing bowl, add baby spinach, shallots, apricots, frisee lettuce.
- ❖ Prepare the vinaigrette by taking a bowl and whisking in all blood orange vinaigrette Ingredients: listed above.
- ❖ Before serving, dress the salad with the prepared orange vinaigrette and toss well.
- ❖ Add fried pita chips and almonds and toss again.
- ❖ Serve into individual bowls with a garnish of two blood orange slices.
- ❖ Enjoy!

Nutrition: Calories: 462, Total Fat: 41.2 g, Saturated Fat: 6.9 g, Cholesterol: 0 mg, Sodium: 110 mg, Total Carbohydrate: 22.6 g, Dietary Fiber: 6.8 g, Total Sugars:

6.8 g, Protein: 6.1 g, Vitamin D: 0 mcg, Calcium: 163 mg, Iron: 3 mg, Potassium: 702 mg

160) EASY TORTELLINI LASAGNA SOUP

Cooking Time: 6 Hours	**Servings:** 6

Ingredients	Ingredients	Directions
✓ 1 lb extra lean ground beef ✓ 1 package (16 oz) frozen cheese filled tortellini ✓ 3 cups beef broth ✓ 1/2 cup yellow onion, chopped ✓ 2 cloves garlic, minced ✓ 1 can (28 oz) crushed tomatoes ✓ 1 can (14.5 oz) petite diced tomatoes ✓ 1 can (6 oz) tomato paste ✓ 1 can (10.75 oz) tomato condensed soup	✓ 1 tsp white sugar ✓ 1 ½ tsp dried basil ✓ 1 tsp Italian seasoning ✓ 1/2 tbsp salt, to taste ✓ 1/4 tsp pepper ✓ Optional: ✓ 4 tbsp fresh parsley ✓ 1/2 tsp fennel seeds ✓ Toppings: ✓ Freshly grated Parmesan cheese ✓ Large spoonful of ricotta cheese	❖ In a large skillet over medium heat, brown the ground beef until cooked through ❖ Add the onion and garlic in the last few minutes of the cooking ❖ While the beef is cooking, pour in the crushed tomatoes, petite diced tomatoes, tomato paste, and tomato condensed soup in the slow cooker. - Don't drain the cans! ❖ Add in the sugar, the dried basil, fennel, Italian seasoning, salt, and pepper, adjust to taste ❖ Stir in the cooked ground beef with onions and garlic ❖ Add in the beef broth – or dissolved beef bouillon cubes into boiling water ❖ Cook on high for 3-4 hours or low for 5-hours. ❖ 15-20 minutes before you are ready to serve the soup, add in the frozen tortellini ❖ Set the slow cooker to high and allow the tortellini to heat through ❖ Allow to cool, then distribute the soup into the container and store in the fridge for up to 3 days ❖ To Serve: Reheat in the microwave or on the stove top, top with freshly grated Parmesan cheese, a large spoonful of ricotta cheese, extra seasonings and freshly chopped parsley.

161) GREEK-STYLE QUINOA BOWLS

Cooking Time: 12 Minutes	**Servings:** 2

Ingredients	Ingredients	Directions
✓ 1 cup quinoa ✓ 1 ½ cups water ✓ 1 cup chopped green bell pepper ✓ 1 cup chopped red bell pepper ✓ 1/3 cup crumbled feta cheese ✓ 1/4 cup extra virgin olive oil	✓ 2-3 tbsp apple cider vinegar ✓ Salt, to taste ✓ Pepper, to taste ✓ 1-2 tbsp fresh parsley ✓ To Serve: ✓ Hummus ✓ Pita wedges ✓ Olives ✓ Fresh tomatoes ✓ Sliced or chopped avocado ✓ Lemon wedges	❖ Rinse and drain the quinoa using a mesh strainer or sieve. Place a medium saucepan to medium heat and lightly toast the quinoa to remove any excess water. Stir as it toasts for just a few minutes, to add a nuttiness and fluff to the quinoa ❖ Then add the water, set burner to high, and bring to a boil. ❖ Once boiling, reduce heat to low and simmer, covered with the lid slightly ajar, for 12-1minutes or until quinoa is fluffy and the liquid have been absorbed ❖ In the meantime, mix whisk together olive oil, apple cider vinegar, salt, and pepper to make the dressing, store in the fridge until ready to serve ❖ Add in the red bell peppers, green bell peppers, and parsley ❖ Give the quinoa a little fluff with a fork, remove from the pot ❖ Allow to cool completely ❖ Distribute among the containers, store for 2-3 days ❖ To Serve: Reheat in the microwave for 1-2 minutes or until heated through. ❖ Pour the dressing over the quinoa bowl, toss add the feta cheese. Season with additional salt and pepper to taste, if desired. Enjoy!

Nutrition: Calories:645;Carbs: 61g;Total Fat: 37g;Protein: 16g

162) SPECIAL SALMON STEW

	Cooking Time: 20 Minutes	Servings: 2

Ingredients		Directions
✓ 1 pound salmon fillet, sliced ✓ 1 onion, chopped ✓ Salt, to taste	✓ 1 tbsp butter, melted ✓ 1 cup fish broth ✓ ½ tsp red chili powder	❖ Season the salmon fillets with salt and red chili powder. ❖ Put butter and onions in a skillet and sauté for about 3 minutes. ❖ Add seasoned salmon and cook for about 2 minutes on each side. ❖ Add fish broth and secure the lid. ❖ Cook for about 7 minutes on medium heat and open the lid. ❖ Dish out and serve immediately. ❖ Transfer the stew in a bowl and keep aside to cool for meal prepping. Divide the mixture into 2 containers. Cover the containers and refrigerate for about 2 days. Reheat in the microwave before serving.

163) BROILED HERB SOLE AND CAULIFLOWER MASHED POTATOES

	Cooking Time: 16 Minutes	Servings: 4

Ingredients		Directions
✓ 12 ounces cauliflower florets, cut into 1-inch pieces ✓ 1 (12-ounce) Yukon Gold potato, cut into ¾-inch pieces (do not peel) ✓ 2 tbsp olive oil ✓ ¼ tsp kosher salt ✓ 2 tsp olive oil, plus more to grease the pan ✓ 3 tbsp chopped parsley	✓ 3 tbsp chopped fresh dill ✓ 1 tbsp freshly squeezed lemon juice ✓ ½ tsp chopped garlic ✓ 1¼ pounds boneless, skinless sole or tilapia ✓ ¼ tsp kosher salt ✓ 4 lemon wedges, for serving	❖ TO MAKE THE CAULIFLOWER MASHED POTATOES ❖ Pour enough water into a saucepan that it reaches ½ inch up the side of the pan. Turn the heat to high and bring the water to a boil. Add the cauliflower and potatoes, and cover the pan. Steam for 10 minutes or until the veggies are very tender. ❖ Drain the vegetables if water remains in the pan. Transfer the veggies to a large bowl and add the olive oil and salt. Taste and add an additional pinch of salt if you need it. ❖ Once the veggies have cooled, scoop ¾ cup of cauliflower mashed potatoes into each of containers. ❖ TO MAKE THE SOLE ❖ Preheat the oven to the high broiler setting. Line a sheet pan with foil and lightly grease the pan with oil or cooking spray. ❖ Mix the oil, parsley, dill, lemon juice, and garlic in a small bowl. Pat the fish with paper towels to remove excess moisture and place on the lined sheet pan. Sprinkle the salt over the fish, then spread the herb mixture over the fish. Broil for about 6 minutes or until the fish is flaky. If your fish is very thin, broil for 5 minutes. ❖ When everything has cooled, place one quarter of the fish in each of the 4 cauliflower containers. Serve with lemon wedges. ❖ STORAGE: Store covered containers in the refrigerator for up to 4 days.

164) DELICIOUS POACHED SALMON WITH CITRUS FRUITS

	Cooking Time: 40 Minutes	Servings: 4

Ingredients		Directions
✓ 6 cups water ✓ ½ cup freshly squeezed lemon juice ✓ Juice of 1 lime ✓ Zest of 1 lime ✓ 1 sweet onion, thinly sliced ✓ 1 cup celery leaves, coarsely chopped	✓ 1 tbsp fresh dill, chopped ✓ 1 tbsp fresh thyme, chopped ✓ 2 dried bay leaves ✓ ½ tsp black peppercorns ✓ ½ tsp sea salt ✓ 1 (24 ounce salmon side, skinned and deboned, cut into 4 pieces	❖ Take a large saucepan and place it over medium-high heat ❖ Stir water, lemon, lime juice, lem0on juice, lime zest, onion, celery, greens, thyme, dill and bay leaves ❖ Strain the liquid through fine mesh sieve, discard any solids ❖ Pour strained poaching liquid into large skillet over low heat ❖ Bring to a simmer ❖ Add fish and cover skillet, poach for 10 minutes until opaque ❖ Remove salmon from liquid and serve ❖ Enjoy! ❖ Meal Prep/Storage Options: Store in airtight containers in your fridge for 1-3 days

Nutrition: Calories: 248;Fat: 11g;Carbohydrates: 4g;Protein: 34g

165)   LETTUCE WRAPS WITH BEAN

	Cooking Time: 20 Minutes	Servings: 4

✓ 8 Romaine lettuce leaves ✓ ½ cup Garlic hummus or any prepared hummus ✓ ¾ cup chopped tomatoes ✓ 15 ounce can great northern beans, drained and rinsed	✓ ½ cup diced onion ✓ 1 tbsp extra virgin olive oil ✓ ¼ cup chopped parsley ✓ ¼ tsp black pepper	❖ Set a skillet on top of the stove range over medium heat. In the skillet, warm the oil for a couple of minutes. Add the onion into the oil. Stir frequently as the onion cooks for a few minutes. ❖ Combine the pepper and tomatoes and cook for another couple of minutes. Remember to stir occasionally. Add the beans and continue to stir and cook for 2 to 3 minutes. Turn the burner off, remove the skillet from heat, and add the parsley. Set the lettuce leaves on a flat surface and spread 1 tbsp of hummus on each leaf. Divide the bean mixture onto the leaves. Spread the bean mixture down the center of the leaves. ❖ Fold the leaves by starting lengthwise on one side. Fold over the other side so the leaf is completely wrapped. Serve and enjoy!

166)   GREEK-STYLE CHICKEN SHISH KEBAB

	Cooking Time: 10 Minutes	Servings: 6

Ingredients: ✓ ¼ cup olive oil ✓ ¼ cup lemon juice ✓ ¼ cup white vinegar ✓ 2 garlic cloves, minced ✓ 1 tsp ground cumin ✓ 1 tsp dried oregano ✓ ½ tsp dried thyme	✓ ¼ tsp salt ✓ ¼ tsp ground black pepper ✓ 2 pounds boneless and skinless chicken breasts, cut up into 1½inch pieces ✓ 6 wooden skewers ✓ 2 large green or red bell peppers, cut up into 1inch pieces ✓ 12 cherry tomatoes ✓ 12 fresh mushrooms	❖ In a large bowl, whisk in olive oil, vinegar, garlic, lemon juice, cumin, thyme, oregano, salt, and black pepper. Mix well. ❖ Add the chicken to the bowl and coat it thoroughly by tossing it. ❖ Cover the bowl with plastic wrap, refrigerate, and allow it to marinate for 2 hours. ❖ Soak your wooden skewers in water for about 30 minutes. ❖ Preheat grill to medium-high heat and lightly oil the grate. ❖ Remove the chicken from your marinade and shake off any extra liquid. ❖ Discard the remaining marinade. ❖ Thread pieces of chicken with bits of onion, bell pepper, cherry tomatoes, and mushrooms alternating between them. ❖ Cook on grill for 10 minutes each side until browned on all sides. ❖ Chill, place to containers. ❖ Pre-heat before eating. Enjoy!

167)   PAN-FRIED SHRIMP AND SUMMER SQUASH WITH CHORIZO

	Cooking Time: 20 Minutes	Servings: 8

✓ 1 lb large shrimp or prawns, peeled and deveined, tail can remain or frozen frozen, thawed ✓ 7 oz Spanish Chorizo, or mild Chorizo or hot Chorizo, sliced ✓ Extra virgin olive oil ✓ Juice of 1/2 lemon ✓ 1 summer squash, halved then sliced, half moons	✓ 1 small hot pepper such as jalapeno pepper, optional ✓ 1/2 medium red onion, sliced ✓ Fresh parsley for garnish ✓ 3/4 tsp smoked paprika ✓ 3/4 tsp ground cumin ✓ 1/2 tsp garlic powder ✓ Salt, to taste ✓ Pepper, to taste	❖ Pat shrimp dry, then season with salt, pepper, paprika, cumin, and garlic powder, toss to coat, set aside ❖ In a large cast iron skillet over medium-high, add the Chorizo and brown on both sides, about 4 minutes or until the Chorizo is cooked, transfer to a plate ❖ In the same skillet, add a drizzle of extra virgin olive oil if needed ❖ Add the summer squash, and a sprinkle of salt and pepper and sear undisturbed for about 3 minutes on one side. turnover and sear another 2 minutes on the other side until nicely colored, transfer the squash to the plate with Chorizo ❖ In the same skillet, now add a little extra virgin olive oil and tilting to make sure the bottom is well coated ❖ Once heated, add the shrimp and cook, stirring frequently, until the shrimp flesh starts to turn a little pink, but still not quite fully cooked, about 3 minutes ❖ Return the Chorizo and squash to the skillet, toss to combine, cook another 3 minutes or until shrimp is cooked – its pink and the tails turn a bright red. Transfer the shrimp skillet to a large serving platter, allow to cool. Distribute among the containers, store for 2-3 days ❖ To Serve: Reheat on the stove for 1-2 minutes or until heated through. Squeeze 1/2 lemon on top, and sliced red onions and hot peppers.

168) LENTIL WITH ROASTED CARROT SALAD AND HERBS AND FETA

	Cooking Time: 25 Minutes	Servings: 4

Ingredients:

- ¾ cup brown or green lentils
- 3 cups water
- 1 pound baby carrots, halved on the diagonal
- 2 tsp olive oil, plus 2 tbsp
- ½ tsp kosher salt, divided
- 1 tsp garlic powder
- 1 cup packed parsley leaves, chopped
- ½ cup packed cilantro leaves, chopped
- ¼ cup packed mint leaves, chopped
- ½ tsp grated lemon zest
- 4 tsp freshly squeezed lemon juice
- ¼ cup crumbled feta cheese

Directions:

- ❖ Preheat the oven to 400°F. Line a sheet pan with a silicone baking mat or parchment paper.
- ❖ Place the lentils and water in a medium saucepan and turn the heat to high. As soon as the water comes to a boil, turn the heat to low and simmer until the lentils are firm yet tender, 10 to minutes (see tip). Drain and cool.
- ❖ While the lentils are cooking, place the carrots on the sheet pan and toss with 2 tsp of oil, ¼ tsp of salt, and the garlic powder. Roast the carrots in the oven until firm yet tender, about 20 to 25 minutes. Cool when done.
- ❖ In a large bowl, mix the cooled lentils, carrots, parsley, cilantro, mint, lemon zest, lemon juice, feta, the remaining 2 tbsp of oil, and the remaining ¼ tsp of salt. Add more lemon juice and/or salt to taste if needed.
- ❖ Place 1¼ cups of the mixture in each of 4 containers.
- ❖ STORAGE: Store covered containers in the refrigerator for up to 5 days.

Nutrition: Total calories: 2; Total fat: 12g; Saturated fat: 3g; Sodium: 492mg; Carbohydrates: 31g; Fiber: 13g; Protein: 12g

169) PUMPKIN SOUP WITH CINNAMON

	Cooking Time: 1 Hour	Servings: 6

Ingredients:

- 1 small butternut squash, peeled and cut up into 1-inch pieces
- 4 tbsp extra-virgin olive oil, divided
- 1 small yellow onion
- 2 large garlic cloves
- 1 tsp salt, divided
- 1 pinch black pepper
- 1 tsp dried oregano
- 2 tbsp fresh oregano
- 2 cups low sodium chicken stock
- 1 cinnamon stick
- ½ cup canned white kidney beans, drained and rinsed
- 1 small pear, peeled and cored, chopped up into ½ inch pieces
- 2 tbsp walnut pieces
- ¼ cup Greek yogurt
- 2 tbsp freshly chopped parsley

Directions:

- ❖ Preheat oven to 425 degrees F.
- ❖ Place squash in bowl and season with a ½ tsp of salt and tbsp of olive oil.
- ❖ Spread the squash onto a roasting pan and roast for about 25 minutes until tender.
- ❖ Set aside squash to let cool.
- ❖ Heat remaining 2 tbsp of olive oil in a medium-sized pot over medium-high heat.
- ❖ Add onions and sauté until soft.
- ❖ Add dried oregano and garlic and sauté for 1 minute and until fragrant.
- ❖ Add squash, broth, pear, cinnamon stick, pepper, and remaining salt.
- ❖ Bring mixture to a boil.
- ❖ Once the boiling point is reached, add walnuts and beans.
- ❖ Reduce the heat and allow soup to cook for approximately 20 minutes until flavors have blended well.
- ❖ Remove the cinnamon stick.
- ❖ Use an immersion blender and blend the entire mixture until smooth.
- ❖ Add yogurt gradually while whisking to ensure that you are getting a very creamy soup.
- ❖ Season with some additional salt and pepper if needed.
- ❖ Garnish with parsley and fresh oregano.
- ❖ Enjoy!

Nutrition: Calories: 197, Total Fat: 11.6 g, Saturated Fat: 1.7 g, Cholesterol: 0 mg, Sodium: 264 mg, Total Carbohydrate: 20.2 g, Dietary Fiber: 7.1 g, Total Sugars: 4.3 g, Protein: 6.1 g, Vitamin D: 0 mcg, Calcium: 103 mg, Iron: 3 mg, Potassium: 425 mg

170)   CHICKEN CREAM

	Cooking Time: 25 Minutes	Servings: 2

Ingredients	Ingredients	Instructions
✓ ½ small onion, chopped ✓ ¼ cup sour cream ✓ Salt and black pepper, to taste	✓ 1 tbsp butter ✓ ¼ cup mushrooms ✓ ½ pound chicken breasts	❖ Heat butter in a skillet and add onions and mushrooms. ❖ Sauté for about 5 minutes and add chicken breasts and salt. ❖ Secure the lid and cook for about 5 more minutes. ❖ Add sour cream and cook for about 3 minutes. ❖ Open the lid and dish out in a bowl to serve immediately. ❖ Transfer the creamy chicken breasts in a dish and set aside to cool for meal prepping. Divide them in 2 containers and cover their lid. Refrigerate for 2-3 days and reheat in microwave before serving.

171)   CHICKEN DRUMMIES AND PEACH GLAZE

	Cooking Time: 25 Minutes	Servings: 4

Ingredients	Ingredients	Instructions
✓ 2 pounds of chicken drummies, remove the skin ✓ 15 ounce can of sliced peaches, drain the juice ✓ ¼ cup cider vinegar ✓ ½ tsp paprika	✓ ¼ tsp black pepper ✓ ¼ cup honey ✓ 3 garlic cloves ✓ ¼ tsp sea salt	❖ Before you turn your oven on, make sure that one rack is 4 inches below the broiler element. ❖ Set your oven's temperature to 500 degrees Fahrenheit. ❖ Line a large baking sheet with a piece of aluminum foil. Set a wire cooling rack on top of the foil. Spray the rack with cooking spray. ❖ Add the honey, peaches, garlic, vinegar, salt, paprika, and pepper into a blender. Mix until smooth. ❖ Set a medium saucepan on top of your stove and set the range temperature to medium heat. Pour the mixture into the saucepan and bring it to a boil while stirring constantly. ❖ Once the sauce is done, divide it into two small bowls and set one off to the side. With the second bowl, brush half of the mixture onto the chicken drummies. Roast the drummies for 10 minutes. ❖ Take the drummies out of the oven and switch to broiler mode. ❖ Brush the drummies with the other half of the sauce from the second bowl. Again, place the drummies back into the oven and set a timer for 5 minutes. When the timer goes off, flip the drummies over and broil for another 3 to 4 minutes. ❖ Serve the drummies with the reserved sauce and enjoy!

172)   WILD BERRIES COMPOTE AND ORANGE MINT INFUSION

	Cooking Time: 20 Minutes	Servings: 8

Ingredients	Ingredients	Instructions
✓ ½ cup water ✓ 3 orange pekoe tea bags ✓ 3 sprigs of fresh mint ✓ 1 cup fresh strawberries, hulled and halved lengthwise ✓ 1 cup fresh golden raspberries ✓ 1 cup fresh red raspberries	✓ 1 cup fresh blueberries ✓ 1 cup fresh blackberries ✓ 1 cup fresh sweet cherries, pitted and halved ✓ 1-milliliter bottle of Sauvignon Blanc ✓ 2/3 cup sugar ✓ ½ cup pomegranate juice ✓ 1 tsp vanilla ✓ fresh mint sprigs	❖ In a small saucepan, bring water to a boil and add tea bags and 3 mint sprigs. Stir well, cover, remove from heat, and allow to stand for 10 minutes. In a large bowl, add strawberries, red raspberries, golden raspberries, blueberries, blackberries, and cherries. Put to the side. ❖ In a medium-sized saucepan, and add the wine, sugar, and pomegranate juice. Pour the infusion (tea mixture) through a fine-mesh sieve and into the pan with wine. ❖ Squeeze the bags to release the liquid, and then discard bags and mint springs. Cook well until the sugar has completely dissolved; remove from heat. ❖ Stir in vanilla and allow to chill for 2 hours. Pour the mix over the fruits. ❖ Garnish with mint sprigs and serve. Enjoy!

173) BRUSCHETTA AND QUINOA SALAD

Cooking Time: 15 Minutes	Servings: 5

Ingredients		Instructions
✓ 2 cups water ✓ 1 cup uncooked quinoa ✓ 1 (10-ounce) container cherry tomatoes, quartered ✓ 1 tsp chopped garlic ✓ 1¼ cups thinly sliced scallions, white and green parts (1 small bunch)	✓ 1 (8-ounce) container fresh whole-milk mozzarella balls (ciliegine), quartered ✓ 2 tbsp balsamic vinegar ✓ 2 tbsp olive oil ✓ ½ tsp kosher salt ✓ ½ cup fresh basil leaves, chiffonaded (cut into strips)	❖ Place the water and quinoa in a saucepan and bring to a boil. Cover, turn the heat to low, and simmer for minutes. ❖ While the quinoa is cooking, place the tomatoes, garlic, scallions, mozzarella, vinegar, and oil in a large mixing bowl. Stir to combine. ❖ Once the quinoa is cool, add it to the tomato mixture along with the salt and basil. Mix to combine. ❖ Place 1⅓ cups of the mixture in each of 5 containers and refrigerate. Serve at room temperature. ❖ STORAGE: Store covered containers in the refrigerator for up to days.

174) PARMESAN CHICKEN WITH LEMON SPAGHETTI AND ZUCCHINI

Cooking Time: 15 Minutes	Servings: 2

Ingredients		Instructions
✓ 2 packages Frozen zucchini noodle Spirals ✓ 1-1/2 lbs. boneless skinless chicken breast, cut into bite-sized pieces ✓ 1 tsp fine sea salt ✓ 2 tsp dried oregano ✓ 1/2 tsp ground black pepper	✓ 4 garlic cloves, minced ✓ 2 tbsp vegan butter ✓ 2 tsp lemon zest ✓ 2 tsp oil ✓ 1/3 cup parmesan ✓ 2/3 cup broth ✓ Lemon slices, for garnish ✓ Parsley, for garnish	❖ Cook zucchini noodles according to package instructions, drain well ❖ In a large skillet over medium heat, add the oil ❖ Season chicken with salt and pepper, brown chicken pieces, for about 4 minutes per side depending on the thickness, or until cooked through – Work in cook in batches if necessary. Transfer the chicken to a pan ❖ In the same skillet, add in the garlic, and cook until fragrant about 30 seconds. Add in the butter, oregano and lemon zest, pour in chicken broth to deglaze making sure to scrape up all the browned bits stuck to the bottom of the pan ❖ Turn the heat up to medium-high, bring sauce and chicken up to a boil, immediately lower the heat and stir in the parmesan cheese ❖ Place the chicken back in pan and allow it to gently simmer for 3-4 minutes, or until sauce has slightly reduced and thickened up ❖ Taste and adjust seasoning, allow the noodles to cool completely ❖ Distribute among the containers, store for 2-3 days ❖ To Serve: Reheat in the microwave for 1-2 minutes or until heated through. Garnish with the fresh parsley and lemon slices and enjoy!

175) SCALLOPS WITH THREE CITRUS SAUCE

Cooking Time: 15 Minutes	Servings: 4

Ingredients		Instructions
✓ 2 tsp extra virgin olive oil ✓ 1 shallot, minced ✓ 20 sea scallops, cleaned ✓ 1 tbsp lemon zest ✓ 2 tsp orange zest ✓ 1 tsp lime zest	✓ 1 tbsp fresh basil, chopped ✓ ½ cup freshly squeezed lemon juice ✓ 2 tbsp honey ✓ 1 tbsp plain Greek yogurt ✓ Pinch of sea salt	❖ Take a large skillet and place it over medium-high heat ❖ Add olive oil and heat it up ❖ Add shallots and Saute for 1 minute ❖ Add scallops in the skillet and sear for 5 minutes, turning once ❖ Move scallops to edge and stir in lemon, orange, lime zest, basil, orange juice and lemon juice ❖ Simmer the sauce for 3 minutes ❖ Whisk in honey, yogurt and salt ❖ Cook for 4 minutes and coat the scallops in the sauce ❖ Serve and enjoy! ❖ Meal Prep/Storage Options: Store in airtight containers in your fridge for 1-2 days

Nutrition: Calories: 207;Fat: 4g;Carbohydrates: 17g;Protein: 26g

176) STEAMED MUSSELS TOPPED AND WINE SAUCE

Cooking Time: 15 Minutes	Servings: 4

Ingredients:

- ✓ 2 pounds mussels
- ✓ 1 tbsp extra virgin olive oil
- ✓ 1 cup sliced onion
- ✓ 1 cup dry white wine
- ✓ ¼ tsp ground black pepper
- ✓ ¼ tsp sea salt
- ✓ 3 sliced cloves of garlic
- ✓ 2 lemon slices
- ✓ Optional: lemon wedges for serving

❖ Set a large colander in the sink and turn your water to cold.

❖ Run water over the mussels, but do not let them sit in the water. If you notice any shells that are not tightly sealed or are cracked, you need to discard them. All shells need to be closed tightly.

❖ Turn off the water and leave the mussels in the colander.

❖ Set a large skillet on your stovetop and turn your range heat to medium-high. Pour the olive oil into the skillet and allow it to heat up before you add the onion.

❖ Saute the onion for 2 to 3 minutes.

❖ Combine the garlic and cook the mixture for another minute while stirring continuously.

❖ Pour in the wine, pepper, lemon slices, and salt. Stir the ingredients as you bring them to a boil.

❖ Add the mussels and place the lid on the skillet.

❖ Cook the mixture for 3 to 4 minutes or until the shells begin to open on the mussels. It will help to gently pick up the skillet and shake it a couple of times when the mussels are cooking.

❖ If you notice any shells that did not open, use a spoon and discard them.

❖ Scoop the mussels into a serving bowl and pour the mixture over the top.

❖ If you have lemon wedges, place them on the top of the steamed mussels before serving. Enjoy!

Nutrition: calories: 222, fats: 7 grams, carbohydrates: 11 grams, protein: 18 grams.

177) DELICIOUS SPICE POTATO SOUP

Cooking Time: 30 Minutes	Servings: 4-6

Ingredients:

- ✓ 2 tbsp extra virgin olive oil
- ✓ 1 large onion, chopped
- ✓ 2 garlic cloves, crushed
- ✓ 1 pound sweet potatoes, peeled and cut into medium pieces
- ✓ ½ tsp ground cumin
- ✓ ¼ tsp ground chili
- ✓ ½ tsp ground coriander
- ✓ ¼ tsp ground cinnamon
- ✓ ¼ tsp salt
- ✓ 2 cups chicken stock
- ✓ ¼ cup of low-fat crème Fraiche
- ✓ 2 tbsp freshly chopped parsley
- ✓ coriander

❖ Heat olive oil in a large pan over medium-high heat.

❖ Add onions and sauté until slightly browned.

❖ Reduce heat to medium, add garlic, and keep cooking for 2-minutes more.

❖ Add sweet potatoes and sauté for 3-minutes.

❖ Add the remaining spices and season with salt.

❖ Cook for 2 minutes.

❖ Add stock, turn the heat up, and bring the mixture to a boil, stirring occasionally.

❖ Cover and lower heat to a slow simmer.

❖ Cook for 20 minutes until the potatoes are tender.

❖ Remove the pan from the heat.

❖ Take an immersion blender and puree the whole mixture.

❖ Add a bit of water if the soup is too thick.

❖ Check the soup for seasoning.

❖ Ladle the soup into your jars.

❖ Give a swirl of crème Fraiche.

❖ Sprinkle with chopped parsley.

❖ Enjoy!

Nutrition: Calories: 176, Total Fat: 8.4 g, Saturated Fat: 0.8 g, Cholesterol: 0 mg, Sodium: 362 mg, Total Carbohydrate: 24.3 g, Dietary Fiber: 3.8 g, Total Sugars: 1.7 g, Protein: 2 g, Vitamin D: 0 mcg, Calcium: 30 mg, Iron: 1 mg, Potassium: 675 mg

178) DELICIOUS SPICY CAJUN SHRIMP

Cooking Time: 50 Minutes	Servings: 2

✓ 3 cloves garlic, crushed ✓ 4 tbsp butter, divided ✓ 2 large zucchini, spiraled ✓ 1 red pepper, sliced ✓ 1 onion, sliced ✓ 20-30 jumbo shrimp	✓ 1 tsp paprika ✓ dash cayenne pepper ✓ ½ tsp of sea salt ✓ dash red pepper flakes ✓ 1 tsp garlic powder ✓ 1 tsp onion powder	❖ Pass the zucchini through a spiralizer. ❖ Combine the Ingredients: listed under Cajun Seasoning above. ❖ Add oil and 2 tbsp of butter to a pan and allow to heat up over medium heat. ❖ Add onion and red pepper and sauté for minutes. ❖ Add shrimp and cook well. ❖ Place the remaining 2 tbsp of butter in another pan and allow it to melt over medium heat. ❖ Add zucchini noodles and sauté for 3 minutes. ❖ Transfer the noodles to a container. ❖ Top with the prepared Cajun shrimp and veggie mix. ❖ Season with salt and enjoy!

179) PAN-SEARED SALMON

Cooking Time: 20 Minutes	Servings: 4

✓ Salmon fillets (4 @ 6 oz. each) ✓ Olive oil (2 tbsp.) ✓ Capers (2 tbsp.)	✓ Pepper & salt (.125 tsp. each) ✓ Lemon (4 slices)	❖ Warm a heavy skillet for about three minutes using the medium heat temperature setting. ❖ Lightly spritz the salmon with oil. Arrange them in the pan and increase the temperature setting to high. ❖ Sear for approximately three minutes. Sprinkle with the salt, pepper, and capers. ❖ Flip the salmon over and continue cooking for five minutes or until browned the way you like it. ❖ Garnish with lemon slices and serve.

180) PASTA FAGIOLI SOUP

Cooking Time: 1 Hour	Servings: 8

✓ 1 28-ounce can diced tomatoes ✓ 1 14-ounce can great northern beans, undrained ✓ 14 ounces spinach, chopped and drained ✓ 1 14-ounce can tomato sauce ✓ 3 cups chicken broth	✓ 1 tbsp garlic, minced ✓ 8 slices bacon, cooked crisp, crumbled ✓ 1 tbsp dried parsley ✓ 1 tsp garlic powder ✓ 1½ tsp salt ✓ ½ tsp ground black pepper ✓ ½ tsp dried basil ✓ ½ pound seashell pasta ✓ 3 cups water	❖ Take a large stockpot and add the diced tomatoes, spinach, beans, chicken broth, tomato sauce, water, bacon, garlic, parsley, garlic powder, pepper, salt, and basil. ❖ Put it over medium-high heat and bring the mixture to a boil. ❖ Immediately reduce the heat to low and simmer for 40 minutes, covered. ❖ Add pasta and cook uncovered for about 10 minutes until al dente. ❖ Ladle the soup into serving bowls. ❖ Sprinkle some cheese on top. ❖ Enjoy!

181) SPECIAL POMEGRANATE VINAIGRETTE

Cooking Time: 5 Minutes	Servings: ½ Cup

✓ ⅓ cup pomegranate juice ✓ 1 tsp Dijon mustard ✓ 1 tbsp apple cider vinegar	✓ ½ tsp dried mint ✓ 2 tbsp plus 2 tsp olive oil	❖ Place the pomegranate juice, mustard, vinegar, and mint in a small bowl and whisk to combine. ❖ Whisk in the oil, pouring it into the bowl in a thin steam. ❖ Pour the vinaigrette into a container and refrigerate. ❖ STORAGE: Store the covered container in the refrigerator for up to 2 weeks. Bring the vinaigrette to room temperature and shake before serving.

Nutrition: (2 tbsp): Total calories: 94; Total fat: 10g; Saturated fat: 2g; Sodium: 30mg; Carbohydrates: 3g; Fiber: 0g; Protein: 0g

182) GREEN OLIVE WITH SPINACH TAPENADE

Cooking Time: 20 Minutes		**Servings: 1½ Cups**

✓ 1 cup pimento-stuffed green olives, drained ✓ 3 packed cups baby spinach ✓ 1 tsp chopped garlic	✓ ½ tsp dried oregano ✓ ⅓ cup packed fresh basil ✓ 2 tbsp olive oil ✓ 2 tsp red wine vinegar	❖ Place all the ingredients in the bowl of a food processor and pulse until the mixture looks finely chopped but not puréed. ❖ Scoop the tapenade into a container and refrigerate. ❖ STORAGE: Store the covered container in the refrigerator for up to 5 days.

Nutrition: (¼ cup): Total calories: 80; Total fat: 8g; Saturated fat: 1g; Sodium: 6mg; Carbohydrates: 1g; Fiber: 1g; Protein: 1g

183) BULGUR PILAF AND ALMONDS

Cooking Time: 20 Minutes		**Servings: 4**

✓ ⅔ cup uncooked bulgur ✓ 1⅓ cups water ✓ ¼ cup sliced almonds	✓ 1 cup small diced red bell pepper ✓ ⅓ cup chopped fresh cilantro ✓ 1 tbsp olive oil ✓ ¼ tsp salt	❖ Place the bulgur and water in a saucepan and bring the water to a boil. Once the water is at a boil, cover the pot with a lid and turn off the heat. Let the covered pot stand for 20 minutes. ❖ Transfer the cooked bulgur to a large mixing bowl and add the almonds, peppers, cilantro, oil, and salt. Stir to combine. ❖ Place about 1 cup of bulgur in each of 4 containers. ❖ STORAGE: Store covered containers in the refrigerator for up to 5 days. Bulgur can be either reheated or eaten at room temperature.

Nutrition: Total calories: 17 Total fat: 7g; Saturated fat: 1g; Sodium: 152mg; Carbohydrates: 25g; Fiber: 6g; Protein: 4g

184) EASY SPANISH GARLIC YOGURT SAUCE

Cooking Time: 5 Minutes		**Servings: 1 Cup**

✓ 1 cup low-fat (2%) plain Greek yogurt ✓ ½ tsp garlic powder ✓	✓ 1 tbsp olive oil ✓ ¼ tsp kosher salt ✓ 1 tbsp freshly squeezed lemon juice	❖ Mix all the ingredients in a medium bowl until well combined. ❖ Spoon the yogurt sauce into a container and refrigerate. ❖ STORAGE: Store the covered container in the refrigerator for up to 7 days

Nutrition: (¼ cup): Total calories: 75; Total fat: 5g; Saturated fat: 1g; Sodium: 173mg; Carbohydrates: 3g; Fiber: 0g; Protein: 6g.

185) DELICIOUS RASPBERRY RED WINE SAUCE

Cooking Time: 20 Minutes		**Servings: 1 Cup**

✓ 2 tsp olive oil ✓ 2 tbsp finely chopped shallot ✓ 1½ cups frozen raspberries ✓ 1 cup dry, fruity red wine	✓ 1 tsp thyme leaves, roughly chopped ✓ 1 tsp honey ✓ ¼ tsp kosher salt ✓ ½ tsp unsweetened cocoa powder	❖ In a -inch skillet, heat the oil over medium heat. Add the shallot and cook until soft, about 2 minutes. ❖ Add the raspberries, wine, thyme, and honey and cook on medium heat until reduced, about 15 minutes. Stir in the salt and cocoa powder. ❖ Transfer the sauce to a blender and blend until smooth. Depending on how much you can scrape out of your blender, this recipe makes ¾ to 1 cup of sauce. ❖ Scoop the sauce into a container and refrigerate. ❖ STORAGE: Store the covered container in the refrigerator for up to 7 days.

Nutrition: (¼ cup): Total calories: 107; Total fat: 3g; Saturated fat: <1g; Sodium: 148mg; Carbohydrates: 1g; Fiber: 4g; Protein: 1g

186) ANTIPASTO SHRIMP SKEWERS

Cooking Time: 10 Minutes	Servings: 4

Ingredients:

- ✓ 16 pitted kalamata or green olives
- ✓ 16 fresh mozzarella balls (ciliegine)
- ✓ 16 cherry tomatoes
- ✓ 16 medium (41 to 50 per pound) precooked peeled, deveined shrimp
- ✓ 8 (8-inch) wooden or metal skewers

Directions:

- ❖ Alternate 2 olives, 2 mozzarella balls, 2 cherry tomatoes, and 2 shrimp on 8 skewers.
- ❖ Place skewers in each of 4 containers.
- ❖ STORAGE: Store covered containers in the refrigerator for up to 4 days.

Nutrition: Total calories: 108; Total fat: 6g; Saturated fat: 1g; Sodium: 328mg; Carbohydrates: ; Fiber: 1g; Protein: 9g

187) SMOKED PAPRIKA WITH MARINATED CARROTS IN OLIVE OIL

Cooking Time: 5 Minutes	Servings: 4

Ingredients:

- ✓ 1 (1-pound) bag baby carrots (not the petite size)
- ✓ 2 tbsp olive oil
- ✓ 2 tbsp red wine vinegar
- ✓ ¼ tsp garlic powder
- ✓ ¼ tsp ground cumin
- ✓ ¼ tsp smoked paprika
- ✓ ⅛ tsp red pepper flakes
- ✓ ¼ cup chopped parsley
- ✓ ¼ tsp kosher salt

Directions:

- ❖ Pour enough water into a saucepan to come ¼ inch up the sides. Turn the heat to high, bring the water to a boil, add the carrots, and cover with a lid. Steam the carrots for 5 minutes, until crisp tender.
- ❖ After the carrots have cooled, mix with the oil, vinegar, garlic powder, cumin, paprika, red pepper, parsley, and salt.
- ❖ Place ¾ cup of carrots in each of 4 containers.
- ❖ STORAGE: Store covered containers in the refrigerator for up to 5 days.

Nutrition: Total calories: 109; Total fat: 7g; Saturated fat: 1g; Sodium: 234mg; Carbohydrates: 11g; Fiber: 3g; Protein: 2g

188) GREEK TZATZIKI SAUCE

Cooking Time: 15 Minutes	Servings: 2½ Cups

Ingredients:

- ✓ 1 English cucumber
- ✓ 2 cups low-fat (2%) plain Greek yogurt
- ✓ 1 tbsp olive oil
- ✓ 2 tsp freshly squeezed lemon juice
- ✓ ½ tsp chopped garlic
- ✓ ½ tsp kosher salt
- ✓ ⅛ tsp freshly ground black pepper
- ✓ 2 tbsp chopped fresh dill
- ✓ 2 tbsp chopped fresh mint

Directions:

- ❖ Place a sieve over a medium bowl. Grate the cucumber, with the skin, over the sieve. Press the grated cucumber into the sieve with the flat surface of a spatula to press as much liquid out as possible.
- ❖ In a separate medium bowl, place the yogurt, oil, lemon juice, garlic, salt, pepper, dill, and mint and stir to combine.
- ❖ Press on the cucumber one last time, then add it to the yogurt mixture. Stir to combine. Taste and add more salt and lemon juice if necessary.
- ❖ Scoop the sauce into a container and refrigerate.
- ❖ STORAGE: Store the covered container in the refrigerator for up to days.

Nutrition: (¼ cup): Total calories: 51; Total fat: 2g; Saturated fat: 1g; Sodium: 137mg; Carbohydrates: 3g; Fiber: <1g; Protein: 5g

Chapter 4. THE BEST RECIPES

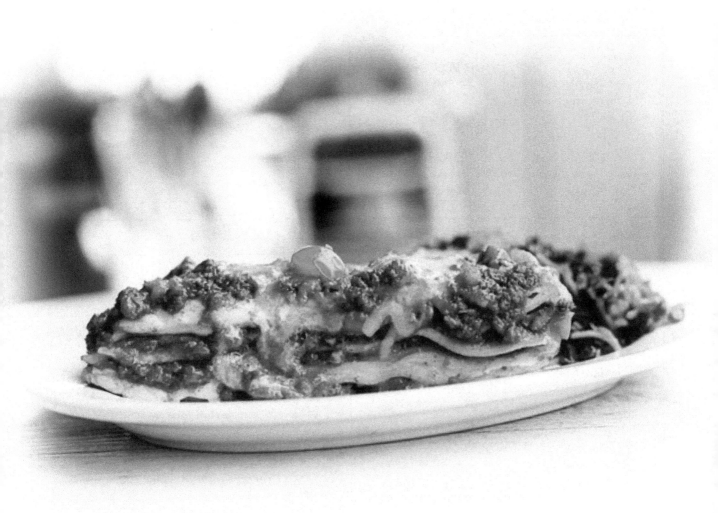

189) ITALIAN BAKED ZUCCHINI WITH THYME AND PARMESAN

Preparation Time: 10 minutes	Cooking Time: 20 minutes	Servings: 4

Ingredients:

- ✓ Four sliced zucchinis
- ✓ 1/2 tsp dried thyme
- ✓ 1/2 cup shredded Parmesan cheese
- ✓ 1/2 tsp dried oregano
- ✓ 2 tbsp olive oil
- ✓ 1/4 tsp garlic powder
- ✓ Kosher salt to taste
- ✓ 1/2 tsp dried basil
- ✓ Black pepper to taste
- ✓ 2 tbsp chopped parsley

Directions:

- ❖ Mix all the ingredients in a large bowl except zucchini.
- ❖ Make a layer of zucchini over a baking sheet sprayed with oil.
- ❖ Transfer the cheese mixture over zucchini and pour olive oil over them.
- ❖ Bake in a preheated oven at 350 degrees for 15 minutes, followed by broiling for three minutes.
- ❖ Serve and enjoy it.

190) ITALIAN BABA GANOUSH

Preparation Time: 10 minutes	Cooking Time: 40 minutes	Servings: 4

Ingredients:

- ✓ One eggplant
- ✓ 1 tbsp Greek yogurt
- ✓ olive oil
- ✓ 1.5 tbsp tahini paste
- ✓ 1 tbsp lime juice
- ✓ One garlic clove
- ✓ Salt to taste
- ✓ 1 tsp cayenne pepper
- ✓ Pepper to taste
- ✓ ½ tsp sumac for garnishing
- ✓ Parsley leaves for garnishing
- ✓ Toasted pine nuts for garnishing

Directions:

- ❖ Make slits in eggplant's skin.
- ❖ Place eggplant skin side upwards in a baking tray.
- ❖ Spray olive oil over eggplant.
- ❖ Bake in a preheated oven at 425 degrees for 40 minutes.
- ❖ Scoop the inner flesh of eggplant out and shift in a food processor. Add garlic, cayenne, yogurt, lime juice, salt, tahini, sumac, pepper, and blend. The baba ganoush is ready.
- ❖ You can refrigerator for better results for 60 minutes and sprinkle oil, sumac, parsley, and nuts and serve.

191) SICILIAN SALMON FISH STICKS

Preparation Time: 10 minutes	Cooking Time: 18 minutes	Servings: 4

- ✓ Fish Sticks
- ✓ 2 lb salmon fillet
- ✓ 1/4 tsp salt
- ✓ 1/4 tsp black pepper
- ✓ First coating
- ✓ 1/2 tsp garlic powder
- ✓ 1/2 tsp dried thyme
- ✓ 1 cup almond meal
- ✓ 1/2 tsp sea salt
- ✓ 1/4 tsp black pepper
- ✓ Second coating
- ✓ 1/2 tsp salt
- ✓ 2/3 cup chickpea flour
- ✓ Third coating
- ✓ Two eggs
- ✓ Dipping Sauce
- ✓ 1/4 tsp salt
- ✓ 1/4 cup Greek yogurt
- ✓ 1 tsp lemon juice
- ✓ 1 tbsp Dijon mustard
- ✓ 1/2 tsp dill
- ✓ 1/8 tsp garlic powder

Directions:

- ❖ Whisk all the ingredients for the dipping sauce list in a bowl and set aside. The dipping sauce is ready.
- ❖ Mix garlic, thyme, and almond meal in a bowl. The first coating is ready.
- ❖ Add chickpea flour in another bowl. The second coating is ready.
- ❖ Beat the eggs in another bowl. Set aside.
- ❖ Sprinkle pepper and salt over sliced fish with removed skin.
- ❖ First, coat the fish with chickpea flour, followed by coating with egg and almond meal coating.
- ❖ Aline coated fish pieces in a baking sheet covered with parchment paper.
- ❖ Bake in a preheated oven at 400 degrees for 18 minutes.
- ❖ Serve baked fish with dipping sauce and serve.

Nutrition: Calories: 92 kcal Fat: 5.7 g Protein: 14.4 g Carbs: 4.5 g Fiber: 1.3 g

192) AFRICAN BAKED FALAFEL

Preparation Time: 10 minutes	Cooking Time: 24 minutes	Servings: 15 patties

Ingredients:

- ✓ 15 oz chickpeas
- ✓ Three cloves garlic
- ✓ 1/4 cup chopped onion
- ✓ 1/2 cup parsley
- ✓ 2 tsp lemon juice
- ✓ 1/2 tsp baking soda
- ✓ 1 tbsp olive oil
- ✓ 1 tsp ground cumin
- ✓ 3/4 tsp salt
- ✓ 1 tsp coriander
- ✓ One pinch of cayenne
- ✓ 3 tbsp oat flour

Directions:

- ❖ Blend all the ingredients except oat flour and baking soda in a food processor to get roughly a blended mixture.
- ❖ Transfer the mixture to a bowl and add oat flour and baking soda. Using hands, mix the dough well.
- ❖ Make patties out of the falafel mixture and set aside for 15 minutes.
- ❖ Bake the falafel patties in a preheated oven at 375 degrees for 12 minutes and serve.

Nutrition: Calories: 143 kcal Fat: 5 g Protein: 6 g Carbs: 24 g Fiber: 6 g

193) GREEK CHIA YOGURT PUDDING

Preparation Time: 10 minutes	Cooking Time: 0 minute	Servings: 4

Ingredients:

- ✓ 3/4 cup milk
- ✓ 11 oz f Vanilla Yogurt
- ✓ 2 tbsp pure maple syrup
- ✓ 1 tsp vanilla extract
- ✓ 1/8 tsp salt
- ✓ 1/4 cup chia seeds
- ✓ Sliced almonds for garnishing

Directions:

- ❖ Whisk all the ingredients in a large bowl. Set aside for 24 hours in the refrigerator.
- ❖ Mix the mixture gently after 24 hours and serve after garnishing.

Nutrition: Calories: 179 kcal Fat: 5.6 g Protein: 10.1 g Carbs: 22.3 g Fiber: 6 g

194) EASY ITALIAN-STYLE FARFALLE

Preparation Time: 10 minutes	Cooking Time: 15 minutes	Servings: 7

Ingredients:

- ✓ 12 oz farfalle pasta
- ✓ ½ cup olive oil
- ✓ ¼ cup chopped basil leaves
- ✓ 1 lb crumbled chorizo sausage
- ✓ ½ cup pine nuts
- ✓ ½ cup shredded parmesan cheese
- ✓ Two chopped garlic cloves
- ✓ 1 cup diced tomato
- ✓ ¼ cup red wine vinegar

Directions:

- ❖ In a saucepan, boil water with added salt.
- ❖ Add pasta and cook until pasta is done.
- ❖ In a pan, cook chorizo over medium flame. Stir in nuts and cook for five minutes.
- ❖ Mix garlic and cook for a minute before removing the pan from the flame.
- ❖ Transfer cooked pasta, vinegar, cheese, cooked chorizo mixture, olive oil, tomatoes, and basil. Mix well to coat everything and serve.

Nutrition: Calories: 692 kcal Fat: 48 g Protein: 26.9 g Carbs: 39.7 g Fiber: 15 g

195) SPECIAL POTATO WEDGES

Preparation Time: 5 minutes	Cooking Time: 30 minutes	Servings: 4

Ingredients:

- ✓ Two wedges cut potatoes
- ✓ ½ tsp salt
- ✓ ½ tsp paprika
- ✓ 1.5 tbsp olive oil
- ✓ ½ tsp chili powder
- ✓ 1/8 black pepper

Directions:

- ❖ Combine all the ingredients in a bowl.
- ❖ Transfer the mixture to an air fryer basket and cook in a preheated air fryer at 400 degrees for eight minutes from both sides.
- ❖ Serve and enjoy it.

196) ORIGINAL GREEK-STYLE POTATOES

Preparation Time: 20 minutes	Cooking Time: 120 minutes	Servings: 4

Ingredients:

- ✓ 1/3 cup olive oil
- ✓ Two chopped garlic cloves
- ✓ 1.5 cups water
- ✓ Black pepper to taste
- ✓ ¼ cup lemon juice
- ✓ 1 tsp rosemary
- ✓ 1 tsp thyme
- ✓ Two chicken bouillon cubes
- ✓ Six chopped potatoes

Directions:

- ❖ Mix all the ingredients in a large bowl and pour over the potatoes placed in the baking tray.
- ❖ Bake in a preheated oven at 350 degrees for 90 minutes.
- ❖ Serve and enjoy it.

197) ORGINIAL ITALIAN-STYLE CHICKEN WRAP

Preparation Time: 10 minutes	Cooking Time: 20 minutes	Servings: 4

Ingredients:

- ✓ 2 tbsp butter
- ✓ 1/2 cup mayonnaise
- ✓ 1/2 lb boneless chicken breasts
- ✓ 1/4 cup shredded Parmesan cheese
- ✓ 2 cups shredded romaine lettuce
- ✓ Four flour tortillas
- ✓ Two sliced Roma tomatoes
- ✓ 1/2 cup crushed croutons
- ✓ 16 basil leaves

Directions:

- ❖ Cook chicken over medium flame in melted butter for 20 minutes.
- ❖ Slice the chicken into strips.
- ❖ Whisk cheese and mayonnaise and pour over the tortilla.
- ❖ Place lettuce followed by chicken, basil, tomato, and croutons on tortilla and wrap.
- ❖ Serve and enjoy it.

198) Lovely Avocado Caprese wrap

Preparation Time: 20 minutes	Cooking Time: 0 minute	Servings: 3

- ✓ Two tortillas
- ✓ Balsamic vinegar as needed
- ✓ One ball mozzarella cheese grated
- ✓ 1/2 cup arugula leaves
- ✓ One sliced tomato
- ✓ 2 tbsp basil leaves
- ✓ Kosher salt to taste
- ✓ One sliced avocado
- ✓ Olive oil as required
- ✓ Black pepper to taste

Directions:

- ❖ Place tomato slices and cheese, followed by avocado and basil. Over one side of the tortilla.
- ❖ Pour olive oil and vinegar. Drizzle pepper and salt.
- ❖ Wrap the tortilla and serve.

199) DELICIOUS CHICKEN SALAD WITH AVOCADO AND GREEK YOGURT

Preparation Time: 10 minutes	Cooking Time: 0 minute	Servings: 4

Ingredients:

- ✓ 1 cup plain yogurt
- ✓ 1 tbsp lemon juice
- ✓ One mashed avocado
- ✓ 1/3 cup dried cranberries
- ✓ Kosher salt to taste
- ✓ 2 cups shredded chicken
- ✓ Black pepper to taste
- ✓ 3/4 cup chopped celery
- ✓ 1/3 cup chopped pecans
- ✓ 1/2 cup chopped red grapes
- ✓ 1/3 cup chopped red onion
- ✓ 2 tbsp chopped tarragon

Directions:

- ❖ Whisk all the ingredients in a large mixing bowl.
- ❖ Serve as a salad and enjoy it.

200) EASY CHICKEN SHAWARMA PITAS

Preparation Time: 10 minutes	Cooking Time: 30 minutes	Servings: 6

- ✓ ¾ tbsp cumin
- ✓ ¾ tbsp coriander
- ✓ ¾ tbsp turmeric powder
- ✓ One sliced onion
- ✓ ¾ tbsp garlic powder
- ✓ ½ tsp cloves
- ✓ ¾ tbsp paprika
- ✓ 1 tbsp lemon juice
- ✓ ½ tsp cayenne pepper
- ✓ Eight boneless chicken
- ✓ Salt to taste
- ✓ 1/3 cup olive oil
- ✓ Pita bread
- ✓ Tahini sauce

Directions:

- ❖ In a bowl, add sliced chicken pieces, onions, cumin, garlic, cloves, olive oil, turmeric, paprika, lemon juice, salt, and coriander. Toss well to coat chicken evenly. Set aside for three hours in the refrigerator.
- ❖ Transfer the chicken pieces along with the marinade in a baking tray sprayed with oil.
- ❖ Bake in a preheated oven at 425 degrees for 30 minutes.
- ❖ Spread tahini sauce in pita bread and add baked chicken pieces. You can also add your favorite salad.
- ❖ Serve and enjoy it.

201) SIMPLE RED LENTIL SOUP

Preparation Time: 10 minutes	Cooking Time: 45 minutes	Servings: 4

- ✓ Four minced garlic cloves
- ✓ ¼ cup olive oil
- ✓ 1 tsp curry powder
- ✓ Two chopped carrots
- ✓ 2 tsp ground cumin
- ✓ One chopped onion
- ✓ ½ tsp dried thyme
- ✓ 1 cup brown lentils
- ✓ 28 oz diced tomatoes
- ✓ 4 cups vegetable broth
- ✓ 1 tsp salt
- ✓ 2 cups of water
- ✓ One pinch of red pepper flakes
- ✓ 1 cup chopped kale
- ✓ Black pepper to taste
- ✓ 1.5 tbsp lemon juice

Directions:

- ❖ Cook carrots and onions in ¼ cup of heated olive oil in a Dutch oven over medium flame for five minutes.
- ❖ Stir in thyme, cumin, garlic, and curry powder,
- ❖ Cook for half a minute.
- ❖ Add tomatoes and cook for another five minutes.
- ❖ Add pepper flakes, broth, salt, lentils, black pepper, and water in a Dutch oven.
- ❖ Let it boil. Cover the oven and lower the flame and let it simmer for 30 minutes.
- ❖ Blend a portion of soup of about two cups in a food processor and transfer it into the pot again.
- ❖ Mix chopped greens and cook for another five minutes.
- ❖ Remove from the flame and mix lemon juice and serve.

Nutrition: Calories: 366 kcal Fat: 15.5 g Protein: 14.5 g Carbs: 47.8 g Fiber: 10.8 g

202) EASY SALMON SOUP

Preparation Time: 10 minutes	Cooking Time: 12 minutes	Servings: 4

Ingredients:

- ✓ Olive oil
- ✓ ½ chopped green bell pepper
- ✓ Four chopped green onions
- ✓ Four minced garlic cloves
- ✓ 5 cups chicken broth
- ✓ 1 oz chopped dill
- ✓ 1 lb sliced gold potatoes
- ✓ 1 tsp dry oregano
- ✓ One sliced carrot
- ✓ ¾ tsp coriander
- ✓ Kosher salt to taste
- ✓ ½ tsp cumin
- ✓ Black pepper to taste
- ✓ Zest of one lemon
- ✓ 1 lb sliced salmon fillet
- ✓ 1 tbsp lemon juice

Directions:

- ❖ Cook onions, garlic, and bell pepper in heated olive oil in a pot over medium flame for four minutes.
- ❖ Stir in the dill and cook for half a minute.
- ❖ Pour broth into the pot. Add carrot, potatoes, salt, spices, and pepper.
- ❖ Let it boil. Reduce the flame and let it simmer for six minutes.
- ❖ Add salmon and cook for five more minutes.
- ❖ Add lemon juice and zest and cook for one minute.
- ❖ Serve the soup and enjoy it.

203) RICH FALAFEL SANDWICHES

Preparation Time: 20 minutes	Cooking Time: 10 minutes	Servings: 4 sandwiches

Ingredients:

- ✓ 4 Pita Breads
- ✓ 1 cup arugula
- ✓ 1 tbsp lemon
- ✓ 1/2 cup tahini sauce
- ✓ 12 falafels
- ✓ One sliced red onion
- ✓ 1/2 cup tabbouleh salad
- ✓ Three sprigs mint

Directions:

- ❖ Spread tahini sauce followed by the addition of arugula and crushed falafels over pita bread.
- ❖ Add tabbouleh salad, mint, and onions over pita and drizzle lemon juice.
- ❖ Wrap the pita bread and serve.

204) EASY ROASTED TOMATO AND BASIL SOUP

Preparation Time: 10 minutes	Cooking Time: 50 minutes	Servings: 6

Ingredients:

- ✓ 3 lb halved Roma tomatoes
- ✓ Olive oil
- ✓ Two chopped carrots
- ✓ Salt to taste
- ✓ Two chopped yellow onions
- ✓ Black pepper to taste
- ✓ Five minced garlic cloves
- ✓ 2 oz basil leaves
- ✓ 1 cup crushed tomatoes
- ✓ Three thyme sprigs
- ✓ 1 tsp dry oregano
- ✓ 2 tsp thyme leaves
- ✓ ½ tsp paprika
- ✓ 2.5 cups water
- ✓ ½ tsp cumin
- ✓ 1 tbsp lime juice

Directions:

- ❖ Mix salt, olive oil, carrot, black pepper, and tomatoes in a bowl.
- ❖ Transfer carrot mixture to a baking tray and bake in a preheated oven at 450 degrees for 30 minutes.
- ❖ Blend baked tomato mixture in a blender. You can use a little water if needed during blending.
- ❖ Sauté onions in heated olive oil over medium flame in a pot for three minutes.
- ❖ Mix garlic and cook for one more minute.
- ❖ Transfer the blended tomato mixture to the pot, followed by the addition of crushed tomatoes, water, spices, thyme, salt, basil, and pepper.
- ❖ Let it boil. Reduce the flame and simmer for 20 minutes.
- ❖ Drizzle lemon juice and serve.

205) GREEK-STYLE BLACK-EYED PEAS STEW

Preparation Time: 5 minutes	Cooking Time: 55 minutes	Servings: 6

- ✓ Olive oil
- ✓ Four chopped garlic cloves
- ✓ 30 oz black-eyed peas
- ✓ One chopped yellow onion
- ✓ One chopped green bell pepper
- ✓ 15 oz diced tomato
- ✓ Three chopped carrots
- ✓ 1.5 tsp cumin
- ✓ One dry bay leaf
- ✓ 1 tsp dry oregano
- ✓ Kosher salt to taste
- ✓ ½ tsp red pepper flakes
- ✓ ½ tsp paprika
- ✓ Black pepper to taste
- ✓ 1 cup chopped parsley
- ✓ 1 tbsp of lime juice
- ✓ 2 cups of water

❖ Cook garlic and onions in a heated oven in a Dutch oven over medium flame for five minutes with constant stirring.
❖ Stir in tomatoes, pepper, water, spices, bay leaf, and salt.
❖ Let it boil.
❖ Mix black-eyed beans and cook for five more minutes.
❖ Cover the oven and reduce the flame. Simmer for 30 minutes.
❖ Squeeze lemon juice and mix.
❖ Serve and enjoy.

206) GREEK CHICKEN GYROS WITH TZATZIKI SAUCE

Preparation Time: 10 minutes	Cooking Time: 8 minutes	Servings: 4

- ✓ Greek Chicken
- ✓ 1 tbsp lemon juice
- ✓ 1/2 cup plain yogurt
- ✓ 1.25 tsp Italian-spiced salt
- ✓ 2 tbsp extra-virgin olive oil
- ✓ 1 cup Tzatziki sauce
- ✓ Four slices of pita bread
- ✓ Four chopped tomatoes
- ✓ 1/4 sliced red onion
- ✓ Tzatziki Sauce
- ✓ ½ halved cucumber
- ✓ ¾ cup Greek yogurt
- ✓ Two minced garlic cloves
- ✓ 1 tbsp red wine vinegar
- ✓ 1 tbsp chopped dill
- ✓ One pinch of kosher salt
- ✓ One pinch of black pepper

❖ Marinate the chicken by mixing it with lemon juice, salt, and yogurt. Set aside for one hour.
❖ Heat olive oil in a skillet over medium flame.
❖ Add chicken without marinade and cook for five minutes from both sides. Transfer the cooked brown chicken to the plate.
❖ Mix all the ingredients of Tzatziki sauce in a bowl and set aside. The Tzatziki sauce is ready.
❖ Toast pita bread and place Tzatziki sauce, tomatoes, onions, and chicken pieces over pita bread. Wrap and serve.

207) GREEK-STYLE CHICKEN MARINADE

Preparation Time: 5 minutes	Cooking Time: 15 minutes	Servings: 4

Ingredients:

- ✓ 1 lb boneless chicken breasts
- ✓ ¼ cup olive oil
- ✓ ½ tsp black pepper
- ✓ 1/3 cup Greek yogurt
- ✓ Four lemons
- ✓ 2 tbsp dried oregano
- ✓ Five minced garlic cloves
- ✓ 1 tsp kosher salt

Directions:

❖ Mix all the ingredients in a bowl and set aside for three hours.
❖ Preheat the grill and grill chicken and lemon slices for 20 minutes from both sides.
❖ Slice the grilled chicken and serve.

208) ITALIAN STYLE CHICKEN QUINOA BOWL WITH BROCCOLI AND TOMATO

Preparation Time: 10 minutes	Cooking Time: 30 minutes	Servings: 3

Ingredients:

- ✓ Chicken
- ✓ 6 oz boneless chicken breast
- ✓ 1 cup Easy Roasted Feta and Broccoli
- ✓ 1/2 cup olive oil
- ✓ 1/2 tsp kosher salt
- ✓ Zest of one lemon
- ✓ 2 tsp dried oregano
- ✓ 1.5 tbsp lemon juice
- ✓ 1/4 tsp black pepper
- ✓ Two minced garlic cloves
- ✓ 1/2 cup Easy Roasted Tomatoes
- ✓ Quinoa
- ✓ 1 tsp kosher salt
- ✓ 1 cup dried quinoa
- ✓ Feta cheese to taste

Directions:

- ❖ Mix lemon juice, oregano, salt, olive oil, garlic, lemon zest, and pepper in a bowl.
- ❖ Add chicken and toss well. Set aside for one hour.
- ❖ Cook chicken in heat olive oil over medium flame for 15 minutes.
- ❖ Lower the flame and stir in tomatoes and broccoli and cook. Set aside.
- ❖ Add water and salt to a pot and bring it to a boil.
- ❖ Add quinoa and cook for ten minutes.
- ❖ Drain the quinoa and set aside.
- ❖ Add quinoa in a bowl, followed by the addition of chicken and veggies. Sprinkle salt, cheese, oil, and pepper.
- ❖ Serve and enjoy it.

209) EASY CHICKEN PICCATA

Preparation Time: 10 minutes	Cooking Time: 10 minutes	Servings: 4

- ✓ 1.5 lb boneless chicken breasts
- ✓ One lemon
- ✓ 2 tbsp canola oil
- ✓ 1 tsp kosher salt
- ✓ 1 cup chicken broth
- ✓ 1 tsp black pepper
- ✓ 2 tbsp capers
- ✓ 3 tbsp butter
- ✓ 1/3 cup all-purpose flour

Directions:

- ❖ Mix salt, flour, and pepper in a bowl. Coat chicken with the flour mixture. Set aside.
- ❖ Cook chicken pieces in heated butter and canola oil over medium flame for five minutes from both sides. Shift cooked pieces onto the plate.
- ❖ Lower the flame and pour broth and add sliced lemon, butter (1 tbsp), lemon juice, capers, and cook for five minutes.
- ❖ Pour the sauce over chicken pieces and serve with cauliflower or noodles.

210) ITALIAN CHOPPED GRILLED VEGETABLE WITH FARRO

Preparation Time: 5 minutes	Cooking Time: 50 minutes	Servings: 2

- ✓ 1 cup dried farro
- ✓ 1 Portobello mushroom
- ✓ 3 cups vegetable broth
- ✓ One sliced red bell pepper
- ✓ 1/2 sliced red onion
- ✓ 8 oz asparagus
- ✓ One sliced zucchini
- ✓ Olive oil as required
- ✓ 1/4 cup halved Kalamata olives
- ✓ One sliced yellow squash
- ✓ Kosher salt to taste
- ✓ 1-pint Greek yogurt
- ✓ Black pepper to taste
- ✓ 2 tbsp minced cucumber
- ✓ One chopped garlic clove
- ✓ 1 tbsp lemon juice
- ✓ 1 tsp chopped dill
- ✓ 1 tsp chopped mint
- ✓ Red bell pepper hummus
- ✓ 1/8 cup feta cheese

- ❖ In a large pot, add broth and farro. Let it boil over a high flame.
- ❖ Lower the flame to medium and cook for half an hour with occasional stirring.
- ❖ Mix veggies with salt, olive oil, and pepper.
- ❖ Grill the veggies in a preheated grill until marks appear on them. Keep them aside.
- ❖ Whisk cucumber, salt, mint, dill, yogurt, lemon juice, and garlic in a bowl.
- ❖ Make the layers of farro, grilled veggies, hummus, olives, and cheese.
- ❖ Pour yogurt sauce and sprinkle mint and serve.

211) QUICK PORK ESCALOPES IN 30 MINUTES WITH LEMONS AND CAPERS

Preparation Time: 10 minutes	**Cooking Time:** 20 minutes	**Servings: 4**

✓ Four boneless pork chops ✓ 1/4 cup all-purpose flour ✓ Eight sage leaves ✓ kosher salt to taste ✓ 2 tbsp chopped parsley ✓ 4 tbsp butter	✓ 1 tbsp vegetable oil ✓ 1/4 cup capers ✓ 1/2 cup white wine ✓ 1 cup chicken stock ✓ One sliced lemon ✓ 4 tbsp lemon juice ✓ Black pepper to taste	❖ One each pork chops, place two sage leaves on both sides. Set aside. ❖ In a bowl, whisk salt, flour, and pepper. ❖ Coat pork chops with flour. Keep the sage leaves in place. ❖ Melt butter in a skillet over medium flame. ❖ Cook pork chops for five minutes from both sides. ❖ Clean the skillet and melt butter in it. Pour wine and add capers in skillet. Cook to concentrate the wine. Pour stock, lemon slices, and lemon juice. Let it boil for five more minutes. ❖ Place pork in sauce and cook for two minutes. Sprinkle parsley and serve.

212) GREEK-STYLE CHICKEN KEBABS

Preparation Time: 40 minutes	**Cooking Time:** 15 minutes	**Servings: 6**

✓ 1 lb boneless chicken breasts ✓ 1/4 cup olive oil ✓ One sliced red bell pepper ✓ 1/3 cup Greek yogurt ✓ 10 tbsp lemons juice ✓ Four chopped garlic cloves	✓ Zest of one lemon ✓ 2 tbsp dried oregano ✓ 1/2 tsp black pepper ✓ One sliced zucchini ✓ 1 tsp kosher salt ✓ One sliced red onion	❖ Whisk all the ingredients except chicken in a bowl. Add chicken and toss to coat chicken evenly. Set aside four hours for better results. ❖ Thread chicken, zucchini, onion, and bell pepper on the skewers. ❖ Grill the chicken, skewers on a preheated grill for 15 minutes, occasionally turning and basting with marinade.

213) EASY PASTA WITH SHRIMP AND ROASTED RED PEPPERS AND ARTICHOKES

Preparation Time: 10 minutes	**Cooking Time:** 25 minutes	**Servings: 8**

✓ 12 oz farfalle pasta ✓ 1/4 cup butter ✓ 1.5 lb shrimp ✓ Three chopped garlic cloves ✓ 1 cup sliced artichoke hearts ✓ 12 oz roasted and chopped red bell peppers ✓ 2 tbsp lemon juice	✓ 1/2 cup dry white wine ✓ 1/4 cup basil ✓ 1/2 cup whipping cream ✓ 3 tbsp drained capers ✓ 1 tsp grated lemon peel ✓ 3/4 cup feta cheese ✓ 2 oz toasted pine nuts	❖ Boil water in a pot and cook pasta in it. ❖ Drain pasta and set aside. ❖ Melt butter in a skillet over medium flame. Sauté garlic and cook for one minute. ❖ Stir in shrimps and cook for about two minutes. ❖ Mix artichokes, capers, bell pepper, and wine. Let it boil. ❖ Lower the flame and let it simmer for two minutes with occasional stirring. ❖ Add whipping cream, lemon juice, and lemon zest. ❖ Let it boil for five minutes. ❖ Transfer the cooked shrimps over pasta and mix well. ❖ Spread cheese, basil, and nuts and serve.

214) CHICKEN CAPRESE QUICK IN 30 MINUTES

Preparation Time: 10 minutes	Cooking Time: 20 minutes	Servings: 4

- ✓ Two boneless chicken breasts
- ✓ Black pepper to taste
- ✓ 1 tbsp butter
- ✓ 1 tbsp extra virgin olive oil
- ✓ 6 oz Pesto
- ✓ Eight chopped tomatoes
- ✓ Six grated mozzarella cheese
- ✓ Balsamic glaze as needed
- ✓ Kosher salt to taste
- ✓ Basil as required

Directions:

- ❖ Mix salt, sliced chicken, and pepper in a bowl. Set aside for ten minutes.
- ❖ Melt butter in a skillet over medium flame.
- ❖ Cook chicken pieces in melted butter for five minutes from both sides.
- ❖ Remove from the flame. Sprinkle pesto and place mozzarella cheese and tomatoes over chicken pieces.
- ❖ Bake in a preheated oven at 400 degrees for 12 minutes.
- ❖ Garnish with balsamic glaze and serve.

215) SPECIAL GRILLED LEMON CHICKEN SKEWERS

Preparation Time: 10 minutes	Cooking Time: 10 minutes	Servings: 6

Ingredients:

- ✓ Two boneless chicken breasts
- ✓ Seven green onions
- ✓ Four minced garlic cloves
- ✓ Three lemons
- ✓ 1 tbsp dried oregano
- ✓ 1 tsp kosher salt
- ✓ 1/4 cup olive oil
- ✓ 1/2 tsp black pepper

Directions:

- ❖ Whisk salt, lemon juice, olive oil, garlic, lemon zest, black pepper, oregano, and sliced chicken pieces in a bowl. Set aside for four hours.
- ❖ Thread chicken, onions, and lemon slices onto the skewer.
- ❖ Grill chicken skewers for 15 minutes on preheated grill over medium flames with often turning.
- ❖ Serve when chicken is fully cooked.

216) TASTY JUICY SALMON BURGERS

Preparation Time: 10 minutes	Cooking Time: 4 minutes	Servings: 4

- ✓ 1.5 lb sliced salmon fillet
- ✓ 3 tbsp minced green onions
- ✓ 1 tsp coriander
- ✓ 2 tsp Dijon mustard
- ✓ 1/3 cup bread crumbs
- ✓ 1 tsp sumac
- ✓ 1 cup chopped parsley
- ✓ ½ tsp sweet paprika
- ✓ Kosher Salt to taste
- ✓ ¼ cup olive oil
- ✓ ½ tsp black pepper
- ✓ One lemon
- ✓ Toppings
- ✓ One sliced red onion
- ✓ Tzatziki Sauce
- ✓ One sliced tomato
- ✓ 6 oz baby arugula

Directions:

- ❖ Blend mustard and salmon in a blender.
- ❖ Shift the mixture in a container. Add all the spices, parsley, salt, and onions. Mix well and set aside for 30 minutes.
- ❖ Make patties out of salmon mixture and place in a tray.
- ❖ Coat all the patties with bread crumbs from both sides.
- ❖ Fry the patties in heated olive oil over medium flame for five minutes each from both sides.
- ❖ Drizzle lemon juice over the cooked patties.
- ❖ Spread Tzatziki sauce over the bun, followed by the layer of salmon, arugula, onions, and tomatoes. The salmon burgers are ready. Serve and enjoy it.

217) SPECIAL BRAISED EGGPLANT AND CHICKPEAS

Preparation Time: 20 minutes	Cooking Time: 55 minutes	Servings: 6

- ✓ 1.5 lb chopped eggplant
- ✓ Olive Oil
- ✓ Kosher salt
- ✓ One chopped yellow onion
- ✓ One chopped carrot
- ✓ One diced green bell pepper
- ✓ Six minced garlic cloves
- ✓ 1.5 tsp sweet paprika
- ✓ Two dry bay leaves
- ✓ 1 tsp organic coriander
- ✓ ¾ tsp cinnamon
- ✓ 1 tsp dry oregano
- ✓ ½ tsp organic turmeric
- ✓ 28 oz chopped tomato
- ✓ ½ tsp black pepper
- ✓ 30 oz chickpeas
- ✓ Handful parsley and mint for garnishing

Directions:

- ❖ Sauté onions, carrots, and bell peppers in heated olive oil over medium flame for four minutes with constant stirring.
- ❖ Stir in salt, bay leaf, garlic, and spices and cook for one minute.
- ❖ Mix eggplant, chickpeas, tomato, and chickpea liquid.
- ❖ Let it boil for ten minutes.
- ❖ Remove the pan from flame and cover.
- ❖ Now, bake in a preheated oven at 400 degrees for 45 minutes.
- ❖ Sprinkle herbs and serve with any sauce.

218) ITALIAN STYLE TUNA SALAD SANDWICHES

Preparation Time: 5 minutes	Cooking Time: 0 minute	Servings: 4

- ✓ 4 tsp red wine vinegar
- ✓ 4 tsp olive oil
- ✓ Eight bread slices
- ✓ ¼ cup chopped red onion
- ✓ 1/3 cup chopped sun-dried tomatoes
- ✓ ¼ tsp black pepper
- ✓ ¼ cup sliced olives
- ✓ 3 tbsp mayonnaise
- ✓ 2 tsp capers
- ✓ Four lettuce leaves
- ✓ 12 oz tuna

Directions:

- ❖ Mix wine and olive oil.
- ❖ Brush bread from both sides with oil mixture.
- ❖ Mix all the ingredients except lettuce and bread slices in a bowl.
- ❖ Place lettuce on each bread slices brushed with oil. Spread tuna mixture and cover with second bread piece and serve.

219) MOROCCAN-STYLE VEGETABLE TAGINE

Preparation Time: 15 minutes	Cooking Time: 40 minutes	Servings: 5

- ✓ ¼ cup extra virgin olive oil
- ✓ Ten chopped garlic cloves
- ✓ Two chopped yellow onions
- ✓ Two chopped carrots
- ✓ One sliced sweet potato
- ✓ Two sliced potatoes
- ✓ Salt
- ✓ 1 tsp coriander
- ✓ 1 tbsp Harissa spice
- ✓ 1 tsp cinnamon
- ✓ 2 cups tomatoes
- ✓ ½ tsp turmeric
- ✓ ½ cup chopped dried apricot
- ✓ 2 cups cooked chickpeas
- ✓ Handful fresh parsley leaves
- ✓ ½ cup vegetable broth
- ✓ 1 tbsp lemon juice

- ❖ Sauté onions in heated olive oil at high flame for five minutes in a Dutch oven.
- ❖ Stir in veggies, salt, garlic, and spices. Mix well and cook for eight minutes over medium flame with constant stirring.
- ❖ Mix in broth, apricot, and tomatoes and cook for the next ten minutes.
- ❖ Reduce the flame and let it simmer for 25 minutes.
- ❖ Add chickpeas and cook for five minutes.
- ❖ Sprinkle parsley and lemon juice and mix well.
- ❖ Serve and enjoy it.

Nutrition: Calories: 448 kcal Fat: 18.4 g Protein: 16.9 g Carbs: 60.7 g Fiber: 24 g

220) ITALIAN-STYLE GRILLED BALSAMIC CHICKEN WITH OLIVE TAPENADE

Preparation Time: 10 minutes	Cooking Time: 30 minutes	Servings: 2

Ingredients:

- ✓ Two boneless chicken breasts
- ✓ 1/4 cup olive oil
- ✓ 1/4 cup balsamic vinegar
- ✓ 1/8 cup garlic mustard
- ✓ 1.5 tbsp balsamic vinegar
- ✓ Three minced garlic cloves
- ✓ 1 tbsp lemon juice
- ✓ 1 tbsp chopped herbs of choice
- ✓ 1 tsp kosher salt
- ✓ 1/2 tsp black pepper

Directions:

- ❖ Combine garlic, balsamic vinegar, lemon juice, pepper, olive oil, herbs, salt, and mustard in a bowl. Add chicken and toss well to coat chicken.
- ❖ Set aside for three hours.
- ❖ Brush oil over chicken pieces and grill gates.
- ❖ Cook chicken on grill gates for ten minutes from both sides.
- ❖ Occasionally brush the chicken with marinade while grilling it.
- ❖ When marks appear over the chicken, shift the chicken to the grill gate's cooler side and cook there for 12 minutes.
- ❖ Again, shift the chicken to the heated side of the grill gate and cook for ten more minutes.
- ❖ Place the grilled chicken on a plate and cover to keep it warm.
- ❖ Serve and enjoy it.

Nutrition: Calories: 352 kcal Fat: 21 g Protein: 35 mg Carbs: 5 g Fiber: 1 g

221) ITALIAN LINGUINE AND ZUCCHINI NOODLES WITH SHRIMP

Preparation Time: 20 minutes	Cooking Time: 20 minutes	Servings: 6

Ingredients:

- ✓ 2/3 cup extra virgin olive oil
- ✓ 1 lb shrimp
- ✓ Four minced garlic cloves
- ✓ Black pepper to taste
- ✓ 12 oz wheat linguine
- ✓ kosher salt to taste
- ✓ 3 tbsp butter
- ✓ Three zucchinis
- ✓ One lemon zested
- ✓ 1 tsp red chili flakes
- ✓ 3 tbsp lemon juice
- ✓ A handful of chopped parsley
- ✓ 1/2 cup shredded Parmesan cheese

Directions:

- ❖ Add salt, garlic, shrimps, pepper, and olive oil. Toss well to coat evenly. Keep it aside.
- ❖ Pour water into a pot and add salt to it. Let it boil and cook linguine in boiling water. Drain linguine and set aside.
- ❖ Heat olive oil in a skillet over medium heat and cook shrimps in it for three minutes from both sides. Shift the cooked shrimps into the plate.
- ❖ Melt butter in the same pan and sauté garlic, lemon juice, chili flakes, and lemon zest for one minute.
- ❖ Pour in pasta water in another pan and cook for three minutes. Add zucchini noodles and cook for two minutes with constant stirring.
- ❖ Transfer the noodles to the garlic mixture pan. Add linguine and cheese. Toss well.
- ❖ Pour in more of the pasta water to make a sauce of the desired level.
- ❖ Add shrimp, zucchini, salt, and pepper, and mix well.
- ❖ You can spread more cheese if you like.
- ❖ Garnish with parsley and serve.

Nutrition: Calories: 521 kcal Fat: 22 g Protein: 28 g Carbs: 52 g Fiber: 4 g

222) SPANISH CHICKEN SAUSAGE AND SHRIMP WITH RICE

Cooking Time: 30 Minutes	Servings: 4

Ingredients:

- ✓ 4 tsp olive oil, divided
- ✓ 1 (12-ounce) package cooked chicken sausage, sliced
- ✓ 6 ounces uncooked peeled, deveined medium shrimp
- ✓ 1 large green bell pepper, chopped (about 1½ cups)
- ✓ 1 small yellow onion, chopped (about 2 cups)
- ✓ 2 tsp chopped garlic
- ✓ 2 tsp smoked paprika
- ✓ 1 tsp dried thyme leaves
- ✓ 1 tsp dried oregano
- ✓ ½ tsp kosher salt
- ✓ ½ cup quick-cooking or instant brown rice
- ✓ 1 (14.5-ounce) can no-salt-added diced tomatoes in juice
- ✓ 1 cup low-sodium chicken broth
- ✓ 1 medium zucchini, halved vertically and sliced into half-moons

Directions:

- ❖ Heat 2 tsp of oil in a soup pot over medium-high heat. When the oil is shimmering, add the sausage and brown for 5 minutes. Add the shrimp and cook for more minute. Remove the sausage and shrimp, and place them on a plate.
- ❖ Add the remaining tsp of oil to the pot, and when the oil is shimmering, add the bell pepper, onion, and garlic. Sauté until soft, about 5 minutes.
- ❖ Add the sausage, shrimp, paprika, thyme, oregano, salt, rice, tomatoes, and broth to the pot, and stir to combine. Bring to a boil, then cover the pot and turn the heat down to low. Simmer for 15 minutes.
- ❖ After 15 minutes, add the zucchini, return the cover to the pot, and continue to simmer for 5 to 10 more minutes, until the zucchini is crisp-tender and the rice has absorbed most of the liquid.
- ❖ Place about 2 cups of the rice mixture in each of 4 containers.
- ❖ STORAGE: Store covered containers in the refrigerator for up to 5 days.

Nutrition: Total calories: 333; Total fat: 14g; Saturated fat: 3g; Sodium: 954mg; Carbohydrates: 29g; Fiber: 6g; Protein: 26g

223) ITALIAN BROCCOLI, ROASTED RED PEPPER, CHEDDAR, AND OLIVE FRITTATA

Cooking Time: 25 Minutes	Servings: 5

Ingredients:

- ✓ Oil or cooking spray for greasing the pan
- ✓ 8 large eggs
- ✓ ½ cup low-fat (2%) milk
- ✓ 1 tsp smoked paprika
- ✓ 6 ounces broccoli florets, finely chopped (about 2 cups)
- ✓ ½ cup chopped jarred roasted red peppers, drained of liquid
- ✓ ⅓ cup pitted black olives, chopped (or other olive of your choice)
- ✓ ¼ cup shredded sharp Cheddar cheese, plus 2 tbsp

Directions:

- ❖ Preheat the oven to 375°F and rub an 8-inch round cake or pie pan with oil, or spray with cooking spray.
- ❖ Break the eggs into a large mixing bowl. Add the milk and smoked paprika, and whisk until well combined.
- ❖ Add the chopped broccoli, red peppers, olives, and ¼ cup of cheese, and mix.
- ❖ Pour the mixture into the oiled pan and top with the remaining 2 tbsp of cheese. Bake for 20 to 25 minutes.
- ❖ Once the frittata is cool, run a spatula around the sides and slice into pieces.
- ❖ Place 1 slice in each of 5 containers and refrigerate.
- ❖ STORAGE: Store covered containers in the refrigerator for up to 5 days.

Nutrition: Total calories: 193; Total fat: 12g; Saturated fat: 5g; Sodium: 295mg; Carbohydrates: 7g; Fiber: 1g; Protein: 13g

224)	CHUTNEY-DIJON SPECIAL PORK FILLET WITH MUSHROOMS AND SPELT PILAF CABBAGE	
	Cooking Time: 40 Minutes	**Servings:** 2

✓ 8 ounces pork tenderloin (freeze half if you can only find a 1-pound package) ✓ ⅓ cup prepared mango or apricot chutney, plus 1 tbsp ✓ 2 tbsp Dijon mustard ✓ 1 tsp chopped garlic ✓ 2 tsp olive oil ✓ 2 tsp olive oil ✓ 4 ounces mushrooms, sliced	✓ 1 small bunch (about 7 ounces) lacinato or curly kale, ribs removed, leaves roughly chopped ✓ ½ tsp chopped garlic ✓ ⅔ cup farro ✓ ¼ cup dry red wine, such as red zinfandel, merlot, or cabernet ✓ 1¼ cups low-sodium vegetable broth (or chicken broth) ✓ ¼ tsp kosher salt	❖ TO MAKE THE PORK ❖ Remove the tough silver skin from the tenderloin with a sharp knife. ❖ In a small bowl, combine ⅓ cup of chutney and the mustard, garlic, and oil. ❖ Place the pork in a gallon-size resealable bag or shallow dish and rub the chutney mixture over the pork. Marinate for at least 8 hours. ❖ When you're ready to cook, preheat the oven to 0°F and line a sheet pan with a silicone baking mat or foil. ❖ Remove the pork from the marinade and place it on the sheet pan. Discard the marinade. Place the pork in the oven for 10 minutes. Turn it over, rub the remaining 1 tbsp of chutney over the top and sides, and roast for another 8 minutes. (Don't worry if extra marinade burns on the baking mat. The pork will be okay.) ❖ Let the pork cool for at least 10 minutes and slice. ❖ Divide the slices between 2 containers. ❖ TO MAKE THE MUSHROOM AND KALE FARRO PILAF ❖ Heat the oil in a soup pot or Dutch oven over medium-high heat. When the oil is shimmering, add the mushrooms and cook for 4 minutes. ❖ Add the kale and garlic, stir, and cook for another 5 minutes. ❖ Add the farro, stir, and cook for 1 minute. Add the red wine and allow to cook for 1 more minute. ❖ Add the broth and salt, increase the heat to high, and bring to a boil. Once it is boiling, turn the heat down to low, cover, and simmer for 30 minutes, until the farro is tender but still has some bite to it. ❖ After it has cooled, place 1 heaping cup of pilaf in each of the 2 pork containers. Refrigerate. ❖ STORAGE: Store covered containers in the refrigerator for up to 5 days. Freeze farro pilaf for up to 6 months.

Nutrition: Total calories: 677; Total fat: 18g; Saturated fat: 3g; Sodium: 1,041mg; Carbohydrates: 76g; Fiber: 10g; Protein: 48g

225)	DELICIOUS TUNA, CABBAGE, EDAMAME AND STRAWBERRY SALAD	
	Cooking Time: 15 Minutes	**Servings:** 3

✓ 2 (5-ounce) cans light tuna packed in water ✓ 8 tbsp Honey-Lemon Vinaigrette, divided ✓ 3 cups prepackaged kale-and-cabbage slaw ✓ 1 cup shelled frozen edamame, thawed	✓ 2 Persian cucumbers, quartered vertically and chopped ✓ 1¼ cups sliced strawberries ✓ 3 tbsp chopped fresh dill	❖ Place the tuna in a small bowl and mix with 2 tbsp of vinaigrette. ❖ In a large mixing bowl, place the slaw, edamame, cucumbers, strawberries, and dill. Toss to combine. ❖ Place ⅓ cup of tuna in each of containers. Place one third of the salad on top of the tuna in each container to lessen the chance of the salad getting soggy. Spoon 2 tbsp of the remaining vinaigrette into each of 3 separate sauce containers. ❖ STORAGE: Store covered containers in the refrigerator for up to days.

Nutrition: Total calories: 317; Total fat: 18g; Saturated fat: 2g; Sodium: 414mg; Carbohydrates: 22g; Fiber: 9g; Protein: 22g

226) ORIGINAL VEGGIE AVOCADO GREEN GODDESS DIP WITH DIPPERS

	Cooking Time: 10 Minutes	Servings: 4

✓ ½ tsp chopped garlic ✓ 1 cup packed fresh parsley leaves ✓ ½ cup fresh mint leaves ✓ ¼ cup fresh tarragon leaves ✓ ¼ tsp plus ⅛ tsp kosher salt	✓ ¼ cup freshly squeezed lemon juice ✓ ¼ cup extra-virgin olive oil ✓ ½ cup water ✓ 1 medium avocado ✓ 1 (1-pound) bag baby carrots ✓ 2 heads endive, leaves separated	❖ Place the garlic, parsley, mint, tarragon, salt, lemon juice, oil, water, and avocado in a blender and blend until smooth. ❖ Place 4 ounces of carrots and half a head of endive leaves in each of 4 containers. Spoon ¼ cup of dip into each of 4 sauce containers. ❖ STORAGE: Store covered containers in the refrigerator for up to 5 days.

227) ITALIAN BLACK OLIVE BREAD

	Cooking Time: 45 Minutes	Servings: 6

✓ 3 cups bread flour ✓ 2 tsp active dry yeast ✓ 2 tbsp white sugar ✓ 1 tsp salt	✓ ½ cup black olives, chopped ✓ 3 tbsp olive oil ✓ 1¼ cups warm water (about 110 degrees Fahrenheit) ✓ 1 tbsp cornmeal	❖ In a large bowl, combine flour, sugar, yeast, salt, black olives, water, and olive oil. Mix well to prepare the dough. ❖ Turn the dough onto a floured surface and knead well for 5-10 minutes until elastic. ❖ Set dough aside and allow it to rise for about minutes until it has doubled in size. Punch the dough down and knead again for 10 minutes. Allow it to rise for 30 minutes more. ❖ Round up the dough on a kneading board, place upside down in a bowl, and line it with a lint-free, well-floured towel. ❖ Allow it to rise until it has doubled in size again. ❖ While the bread is rising up for the third and final time, take a pan, fill it up with water, and place it at the bottom of your oven. ❖ Preheat oven to a temperature of 500 degrees Fahrenheit. ❖ Turn the loaf out onto a sheet pan, lightly oil it, and dust with cornmeal. ❖ Bake for about 15 minutes. ❖ Reduce heat to 375 degrees Fahrenheit and bake for another 30 minutes. ❖ Cool and chill. ❖ Enjoy!

228) SPECIAL COCOA-ALMOND BLISS BITES

	Cooking Time: 1 Hour	Servings: 10

✓ 1 medium ripe banana, mashed ✓ 3 tbsp ground flaxseed ✓ ½ cup rolled oats ✓ ½ cup plain, unsalted almond butter	✓ 2 tbsp unsweetened cocoa powder ✓ ¼ cup almond meal ✓ ¼ tsp ground cinnamon ✓ 2 tsp pure maple syrup	❖ Combine all the ingredients in a medium mixing bowl. ❖ Roll the mixture into 10 balls, slightly smaller than a golf ball, and place on a plate. ❖ Freeze the bites for 1 hour to harden. ❖ Place 2 bites in each of 5 small containers or resealable bags and store in the refrigerator. ❖ STORAGE: Store covered containers or resealable bags in the refrigerator for up to days. If you want to make a big batch, the bites can be frozen for up to 3 months.

Nutrition: (2 bites): Total calories: 130; Total fat: 9g; Saturated fat: 1g; Sodium: 1mg; Carbohydrates: 11g; Fiber: 3g; Protein: 5g

229) CRUNCHY CRISPBREAD WITH MASCARPONE AND BERRY-CHIA JAM

	Cooking Time: 5 Minutes	Servings: 3

Ingredients:

- ✓ 1 (1-pound) bag frozen mixed berries
- ✓ 2 tsp freshly squeezed lemon juice
- ✓ 2 tsp pure maple syrup
- ✓ 2 tbsp plus 2 tsp chia seeds
- ✓ 6 slices crispbread
- ✓ 3 tbsp mascarpone cheese

Directions:

- ❖ Place the frozen berries in a saucepan over medium heat. When the berries are defrosted, about 5 minutes, mash with a potato masher. You can leave them chunky.
- ❖ Turn the heat off and add the lemon juice, maple syrup, and chia seeds.
- ❖ Allow the jam to cool, then place in the refrigerator to thicken for about an hour.
- ❖ Place 2 slices of crispbread in each of 3 resealable sandwich bags. Place 1 tbsp of mascarpone and 2 tbsp of jam in each of 3 containers with dividers. Alternatively, put the mascarpone and jam in separate small sauce containers.
- ❖ STORAGE: Store crispbread at room temperature and jam and mascarpone in the refrigerator. Mascarpone will last for 7 days in the refrigerator, while jam will last for 2 weeks. Jam can be frozen for up to 3 months.

Nutrition: Total calories: 2; Total fat: 9g; Saturated fat: 3g; Sodium: 105mg; Carbohydrates: 40g; Fiber: 14g; Protein: 6g

230) ZUCCHINI STUFFED WITH SPICY CHICKEN SPECIAL WITH BROWN RICE AND LENTILS

	Cooking Time: 35 Minutes	Servings: 3

- ✓ ⅓ cup long-grain brown rice
- ✓ 1⅔ cups water
- ✓ ⅛ tsp kosher salt
- ✓ ⅓ cup brown lentils
- ✓ 2 tsp olive oil
- ✓ 3 tbsp chopped fresh dill
- ✓ 3 medium zucchini, halved lengthwise and flesh scooped out with a tsp (zucchini flesh reserved)
- ✓ 3 tsp olive oil, divided
- ✓ 1 small yellow onion, chopped
- ✓ 1 tsp chopped garlic
- ✓ ½ pound ground lean chicken
- ✓ ¾ tsp ground cumin
- ✓ ¾ tsp ground coriander
- ✓ ¾ tsp caraway seeds
- ✓ ⅛ tsp red chili flakes
- ✓ 3 tbsp tomato paste
- ✓ ¼ tsp kosher salt
- ✓ ¼ cup feta cheese

- ❖ TO MAKE THE BROWN RICE AND LENTILS
- ❖ Place the rice, water, and salt in a saucepan over high heat. Once the water is boiling, cover the pan and reduce the heat to low. Simmer for 15 minutes.
- ❖ After 15 minutes, add the lentils and stir. Cover the pan and cook for another 15 minutes.
- ❖ If there is a little bit of water still in the pan after the rice and lentils are tender, cook uncovered for a couple of minutes.
- ❖ Stir in the oil and chopped dill.
- ❖ Once the mixture has cooled, place ⅔ cup in each of 3 containers.
- ❖ TO MAKE THE STUFFED ZUCCHINI
- ❖ Preheat the oven to 400°F and line a sheet pan with a silicone baking mat or parchment paper. Place the zucchini boats on a lined sheet pan and coat with 1 tsp of oil.
- ❖ In a 12-inch skillet, heat the remaining 2 tsp of oil over medium-high heat. When the oil is shimmering, add the onion and garlic and cook for 5 minutes. Add the zucchini flesh and cook for 2 more minutes.
- ❖ Add the ground chicken, breaking it up with a spatula. Cook for 5 more minutes.
- ❖ Add the cumin, coriander, caraway seeds, chili flakes, tomato paste, and salt, and cook for another 2 minutes.
- ❖ Mound the chicken mixture into the zucchini boats. Top each zucchini boat with 2 tsp of feta cheese. Bake for 20 minutes.
- ❖ Once cooled, place 2 zucchini halves in each of the 3 rice-and-lentil containers.
- ❖ STORAGE: Store covered containers in the refrigerator for up to 5 days. Brown rice and lentils can be frozen for up to 3 months.

Nutrition: Total calories: 414; Total fat: 19g; Saturated fat: 5g; Sodium: 645mg; Carbohydrates: 39g; Fiber: 10g; Protein: 26g

231) SWEET APPLE, CINNAMON, AND WALNUT BAKED OATMEAL

	Cooking Time: 40 Minutes	**Servings:** 8

Ingredients	Ingredients	Directions
✓ Cooking spray or oil for greasing the pan ✓ 3 small Granny Smith apples (about 1 pound), skin-on, chopped into ½-inch dice ✓ 3 cups rolled oats ✓ 1 tsp baking powder ✓ 3 tbsp ground flaxseed	✓ 1 tsp ground cinnamon ✓ 2 eggs ✓ ¼ cup olive oil ✓ 1½ cups low-fat (2%) milk ✓ ⅓ cup pure maple syrup ✓ ½ cup walnut pieces (if you buy walnut halves, roughly chop the nuts)	❖ Preheat the oven to 350°F and spray an 8-by-inch baking dish with cooking spray or rub with oil. ❖ Combine the apples, oats, baking powder, flaxseed, cinnamon, eggs, oil, milk, and maple syrup in a large mixing bowl and pour into the prepared baking dish. ❖ Sprinkle the walnut pieces evenly across the oatmeal and bake for 40 minutes. ❖ Allow the oatmeal to cool and cut it into 8 pieces. Place 1 piece in each of 5 containers. Take the other 3 pieces and either eat as a snack during the week or freeze for a later time. ❖ STORAGE: Store covered containers in the refrigerator for up to 6 days. If frozen, oatmeal will last 6 months.

Nutrition: Total calories: 349; Total fat: 18g; Saturated fat: 3g; Sodium: 108mg; Carbohydrates: 43g; Fiber: ; Protein: 9g

232) DELICIOUS CHOCOLATE AND PEANUT BUTTER YOGURT WITH BERRIES

	Cooking Time: 15 Minutes	**Servings:** 4

Ingredients	Ingredients	Directions
✓ 2 cups low-fat (2%) plain Greek yogurt ✓ 4 tbsp unsweetened cocoa powder ✓ 4 tbsp natural-style peanut butter	✓ 1 tbsp pure maple syrup ✓ 1 cup fresh or frozen berries of your choice	❖ In a medium bowl, mix the yogurt, cocoa powder, peanut butter, and maple syrup until well combined. ❖ Spoon ½ cup of the yogurt mixture and ¼ cup of berries into each of 4 containers. ❖ STORAGE: Store covered containers in the refrigerator for up to 5 days.

Nutrition: Total calories: 225; Total fat: 12g; Saturated fat: ; Sodium: 130mg; Carbohydrates: 19g; Fiber: 4g; Protein: 16g

233) AUTHENTIC OLIVE FOUGASSE

	Cooking Time: 20 Minutes	**Servings:** 4

Ingredients	Ingredients	Directions
✓ 3 2/3 cups bread flour ✓ 3 1/2 tbsp olive oil ✓ 1 2/3 tbsp bread yeast	✓ 1 1/4 cups black olives, chopped ✓ 1 tsp oregano ✓ 1 tsp salt ✓ 1 cup water	❖ Add flour to a bowl. ❖ Make a well in the center and add the water and remaining Ingredients:. ❖ Knead the dough well until it becomes slightly elastic. ❖ Mold it into a ball and let stand for about 1 hour. ❖ Divide the pastry into four pieces of equal portions. ❖ Flatten the balls using a rolling pin and place it on a floured baking tray. ❖ Make incisions on the bread. ❖ Allow them to rest for about 30 minutes ❖ Preheat oven to 425 degrees Fahrenheit. ❖ Brush the Fougasse with olive oil and allow it to bake for 20 minutes. ❖ Turn the oven off and allow it to rest for 5 minutes. ❖ Remove and allow it to cool. ❖ Enjoy!

234)	**ITALIAN MAPLE-CARDAMOM CHIA PUDDING WITH BLUEBERRIES**	
	Cooking Time: 5 Minutes	Servings: 5

✓ 2½ cups low-fat (2%) milk ✓ ½ cup chia seeds ✓ 1 tbsp plus 1 tsp pure maple syrup	✓ ¼ tsp ground cardamom ✓ 2½ cups frozen blueberries	❖ Place the milk, chia seeds, maple syrup, and cardamom in a large bowl and stir to combine. ❖ Spoon ½ cup of the mixture into each of 5 containers. ❖ Place ½ cup of frozen blueberries in each container and stir to combine. Let the pudding sit for at least an hour in the refrigerator before eating. ❖ STORAGE: Store covered containers in the refrigerator for up to 5 days.

Nutrition: Total calories: 218; Total fat: 8g; Saturated fat: 2g; Sodium: 74mg; Carbohydrates: 28g; Fiber: 10g; Protein: 10g

235)	**DELICIOUS CHEESE BREAD**	
	Cooking Time: 15 Minutes	Servings: 12

✓ 3 cups shredded cheddar cheese ✓ 1 cup mayonnaise ✓ 1 1-ounce pack dry ranch dressing mix	✓ 1 2-ounce can chopped black olives, drained ✓ 4 green onions, sliced ✓ 2 French baguettes, cut into ½ inch slices	❖ Preheat oven to 350 degrees Fahrenheit. ❖ In a medium-sized bowl, combine cheese, ranch dressing mix, mayonnaise, onions, and olives. ❖ Increase mayo if you want a juicier mixture. ❖ Spread cheese mixture on top of your French baguette slices. ❖ Arrange the slices in a single layer on a large baking sheet. ❖ Bake for about 15 minutes until the cheese is bubbly and browning. ❖ Cool and chill. ❖ Serve warm!

Nutrition: Calories: 2, Total Fat: 17 g, Saturated Fat: 7.2 g, Cholesterol: 35 mg, Sodium: 578 mg, Total Carbohydrate: 23.9 g, Dietary Fiber: 1.1 g, Total Sugars: 2.4 g, Protein: 11.1 g, Vitamin D: 3 mcg, Calcium: 229 mg, Iron: 2 mg, Potassium: 85 mg

236)	**DELICIOUS CARROT-CHICKPEA FRITTERS**	
	Cooking Time: 10 Minutes	Servings: 3

✓ 2 tsp olive oil, plus 1 tbsp ✓ 3 cups shredded carrots ✓ 1 (4-ounce) bunch scallions, white and green parts chopped ✓ 1 (15-ounce) can low-sodium chickpeas, drained and rinsed ✓ ⅓ cup dried apricots (about 10 small apricot halves), chopped	✓ 1 tsp garlic powder ✓ 1½ tsp dried mint ✓ ⅓ cup chickpea flour ✓ 1 egg ✓ ¼ tsp kosher salt ✓ 1 tbsp freshly squeezed lemon juice ✓ 1 (5-ounce) package arugula ✓ ¾ cup Garlic Yogurt Sauce	❖ Heat 2 tsp of oil in a -inch skillet over medium-high heat. Once the oil is hot, add the carrots and scallions, and cook for 5 minutes. Allow to cool. ❖ While the carrots are cooking, mash the chickpeas in a large mixing bowl with the bottom of a coffee mug. (I find a coffee mug works better than a potato masher.) ❖ Add the apricots, garlic powder, mint, chickpea flour, egg, salt, lemon juice, and cooked carrot mixture to the bowl, and stir until well combined. ❖ Form 6 patties and place them on a plate. ❖ Heat the remaining 1 tbsp of oil in the same skillet over medium-high heat. Once the oil is hot, add the patties. Cook for 3 minutes on each side, or until each side is browned. ❖ Place 2 cooled fritters in each of 3 containers. Place about 2 cups of arugula in each of 3 other containers, and spoon ¼ cup Garlic Yogurt Sauce into each of 3 separate containers, or next to the arugula. The arugula and sauce are served at room temperature, while the fritters will be reheated. ❖ STORAGE:Store covered containers in the refrigerator for up to 5 days. Uncooked patties can be frozen for 3 to 4 months.

Nutrition: Total calories: 461; Total fat: 17g; Saturated fat: 3g; Sodium: 393mg; Carbohydrates: 61g; Fiber: 15g; Protein: 21g

237) ITALIAN WHOLE-WHEAT PASTA WITH LENTIL BOLOGNESE

Cooking Time: 55 Minutes	**Servings:** 4

- ✓ 2 tbsp olive oil, divided
- ✓ 1 small yellow onion, chopped (about 2 cups)
- ✓ 1 tbsp chopped garlic
- ✓ 2 medium carrots, peeled, halved vertically, and sliced (about 1¼ cup)
- ✓ 8 ounces button or cremini mushrooms, roughly chopped (about 4 cups)
- ✓ 1 tsp dried Italian herbs
- ✓ 2 tbsp tomato paste
- ✓ ½ cup dry red wine
- ✓ 1 (28-ounce) can no-salt-added crushed tomatoes
- ✓ 2 cups water
- ✓ 1 cup uncooked brown lentils
- ✓ ½ tsp kosher salt
- ✓ 8 ounces dry whole-wheat penne pasta
- ✓ ¼ cup nutritional yeast

❖ Heat a soup pot on medium-high heat with tbsp of oil. Once the oil is shimmering, add the onion and garlic, and cook for 2 minutes.

❖ Add the carrots and mushrooms, then stir and cook for another 5 minutes.

❖ Add the Italian herbs and tomato paste, stir to evenly incorporate, and cook for 5 more minutes, without stirring.

❖ Add the wine and scrape up any bits from the bottom of the pan. Cook for 2 more minutes.

❖ Add the tomatoes, water, lentils, and salt. Bring to a boil, then turn the heat down to low and simmer for 40 minutes.

❖ While the sauce is cooking, cook the pasta according to the package directions, drain, and cool.

❖ When the sauce is done simmering, stir in the remaining 1 tbsp of oil and the nutritional yeast. Cool the sauce.

❖ Combine 1 cup of cooked pasta and 1⅓ cups of sauce in each of 4 containers. Freeze the remaining sauce for a later meal.

❖ STORAGE: Store covered containers in the refrigerator for up to 5 days.

Nutrition: Total calories: 570; Total fat: 9g; Saturated fat: 1g; Sodium: 435mg; Carbohydrates: 96g; Fiber: 17g; Protein: 27g

238) ORIGINAL STRAWBERRIES WITH COTTAGE CHEESE AND PISTACHIOS

Cooking Time: 35 Minutes	**Servings:** 5

- ✓ 16 ounces low-fat cottage cheese
- ✓ 16 ounces strawberries, hulled and sliced
- ✓ ½ cup plus 2 tbsp unsalted shelled pistachios

❖ Spoon ⅓ cup of cottage cheese into each of 5 containers.

❖ Top each scoop of cottage cheese with ⅔ cup of strawberries and tbsp of pistachios.

❖ Refrigerate.

❖ STORAGE: Store covered containers in the refrigerator for up to 5 days.

Nutrition: Total calories: 184; Total fat: 9g; Saturated fat: 2g; Sodium: 26g; Carbohydrates: 14g; Fiber: 4g; Protein: 15g

239) SPECIAL TURKEY MEATBALLS WITH TOMATO SAUCE AND ROASTED SPAGHETTI SQUASH

Cooking Time: 35 Minutes	**Servings:** 3

FOR THE SPAGHETTI SQUASH
- ✓ 3 pounds spaghetti squash
- ✓ 1 tsp olive oil
- ✓ ¼ tsp kosher salt

FOR THE MEATBALLS
- ✓ ½ pound lean ground turkey
- ✓ 4 ounces mushrooms, finely chopped (about 1½ cups)
- ✓ 2 tbsp onion powder
- ✓ 1 tbsp garlic powder

- ✓ 1 tsp dried Italian herbs
- ✓ ⅛ tsp kosher salt
- ✓ 1 large egg

FOR THE SAUCE
- ✓ 1 (28-ounce) can crushed tomatoes
- ✓ 1 cup shredded carrots
- ✓ 1 tsp garlic powder
- ✓ 1 tsp onion powder
- ✓ ¼ tsp kosher salt

TO MAKE THE SPAGHETTI SQUASH

❖ Preheat the oven to 4°F and place a silicone baking mat or parchment paper on a sheet pan. Using a heavy, sharp knife, cut the ends off the spaghetti squash. Stand the squash upright and cut down the middle. Scrape out the seeds and stringy flesh with a spoon and discard.

❖ Rub the oil on the cut sides of the squash and sprinkle with the salt. Lay the squash cut-side down on the baking sheet. Roast for 30 to 35 minutes, until the flesh is tender when poked with a sharp knife. When the squash is cool enough to handle, scrape the flesh out with a fork and place about 1 cup in each of 3 containers.

TO MAKE THE MEATBALLS AND SAUCE

❖ Place all the ingredients for the meatballs in a large bowl. Mix with your hands until all the ingredients are combined. Place all the sauce ingredients in an by-11-inch glass or ceramic baking dish, and stir to combine. Form 12 golf-ball-size meatballs and place each directly in the baking dish of tomato sauce. Place the baking dish in the oven and bake for 25 minutes. Cool.

❖ Place 4 meatballs and 1 cup of sauce in each of the 3 squash containers.

240) ITALIAN SALMON CAKES WITH STEAMED GREEN BEAN GREMOLATA

Cooking Time: 6 Minutes		Servings: 4

✓ 2 (6-ounce) cans skinless, boneless salmon, drained ✓ ½ tsp garlic powder ✓ ⅓ cup minced shallot ✓ 2 tbsp Dijon mustard ✓ 2 eggs ✓ ½ cup panko bread crumbs ✓ 1 tbsp capers, chopped ✓ 1 cup chopped parsley	✓ ⅓ cup chopped sun-dried tomatoes ✓ 1 tbsp freshly squeezed lemon juice ✓ 1 tbsp olive oil ✓ Zest of 2 lemons (about 2 tbsp when zested with a Microplane) ✓ ¼ cup minced parsley ✓ 1 tsp minced garlic ✓ ¼ tsp kosher salt ✓ 1 tsp olive oil ✓ 1 pound green beans, trimmed	❖ TO MAKE THE SALMON CAKES ❖ In a large bowl, place the salmon, garlic, shallot, mustard, eggs, bread crumbs, capers, parsley, tomatoes, and lemon juice. Stir well to combine. ❖ Form 8 patties and place them on a plate. ❖ Heat the oil in a 12-inch skillet over medium-high heat. Once the oil is hot, add the patties. Cook for 3 minutes on each side, or until each side is browned. ❖ Place 2 cooled salmon cakes in each of 4 containers. ❖ TO MAKE THE GREEN BEANS ❖ In a small bowl, combine the lemon zest, parsley, garlic, salt, and oil. ❖ Bring about ¼ to ½ inch of water to a boil in a soup pot, Dutch oven, or skillet. ❖ Once the water is boiling, add the green beans, cover, and set a timer for 3 minutes. The green beans should be crisp-tender. ❖ Drain the green beans and transfer to a large bowl. Add the gremolata (lemon zest mixture) and toss to combine. ❖ Divide the green beans among the 4 salmon cake containers. If using, place ¼ cup of Garlic Yogurt Sauce in each of 4 sauce containers. Refrigerate.

241) SPECIAL ITALIAN POPCORN TRAIL MIX

Cooking Time: 35 Minutes		Servings: 5

✓ 12 dried apricot halves, quartered ✓ ⅔ cup whole, unsalted almonds	✓ ½ cup green pumpkin seeds (pepitas) ✓ 4 cups air-popped lightly salted popcorn	❖ Place the apricots, almonds, and pumpkin seeds in a medium bowl and toss with clean hands to evenly mix. ❖ Scoop about ⅓ cup of the mixture into each of 5 containers or resealable sandwich bags. Place ¾ cup of popcorn in each of 5 separate containers or resealable bags. You will have one extra serving. ❖ Mix the popcorn and the almond mixture together when it's time to eat. (The apricots make the popcorn stale quickly, which is why they're stored separately.) ❖ STORAGE: Store covered containers or resealable bags at room temperature for up to 5 days.

242) PORTOBELLO MUSHROOMS STUFFED WITH TYPICAL CREAMY SHRIMPS

Cooking Time: 40 Minutes		Servings: 3

✓ 1 tsp olive oil, plus 2 tbsp ✓ 6 portobello mushrooms, caps and stems separated and stems chopped ✓ 2 tsp chopped garlic ✓ 10 ounces uncooked peeled, deveined shrimp, thawed if frozen, roughly chopped ✓ 1 (14.5-ounce) can no-salt-added diced tomatoes	✓ 1 (14.5-ounce) can no-salt-added diced tomatoes ✓ 4 tbsp roughly chopped fresh basil ✓ ½ cup mascarpone cheese ✓ ¼ cup panko bread crumbs ✓ 4 tbsp grated Parmesan, divided ✓ ¼ tsp kosher salt ✓ 6 ounces broccoli florets, finely chopped (about 2 cups)	❖ Preheat the oven to 350°F. Line a sheet pan with a silicone baking mat or parchment paper. Rub 1 tsp of oil over the bottom (stem side) of the mushroom caps and place on the lined sheet pan, stem-side up. ❖ Heat the remaining 2 tbsp of oil in a 12-inch skillet on medium-high heat. Once the oil is shimmering, add the chopped mushroom stems and broccoli, and sauté for 2 to minutes. Add the garlic and shrimp, and continue cooking for 2 more minutes. Add the tomatoes, basil, mascarpone, bread crumbs, 3 tbsp of Parmesan, and the salt. Stir to combine and turn the heat off. ❖ With the mushroom cap openings facing up, mound slightly less than 1 cup of filling into each mushroom. Top each with ½ tsp of the remaining Parmesan cheese. Bake the mushrooms for 35 minutes. Place 2 mushroom caps in each of 3 containers. ❖ STORAGE: Store covered containers in the refrigerator for up to 4 days.

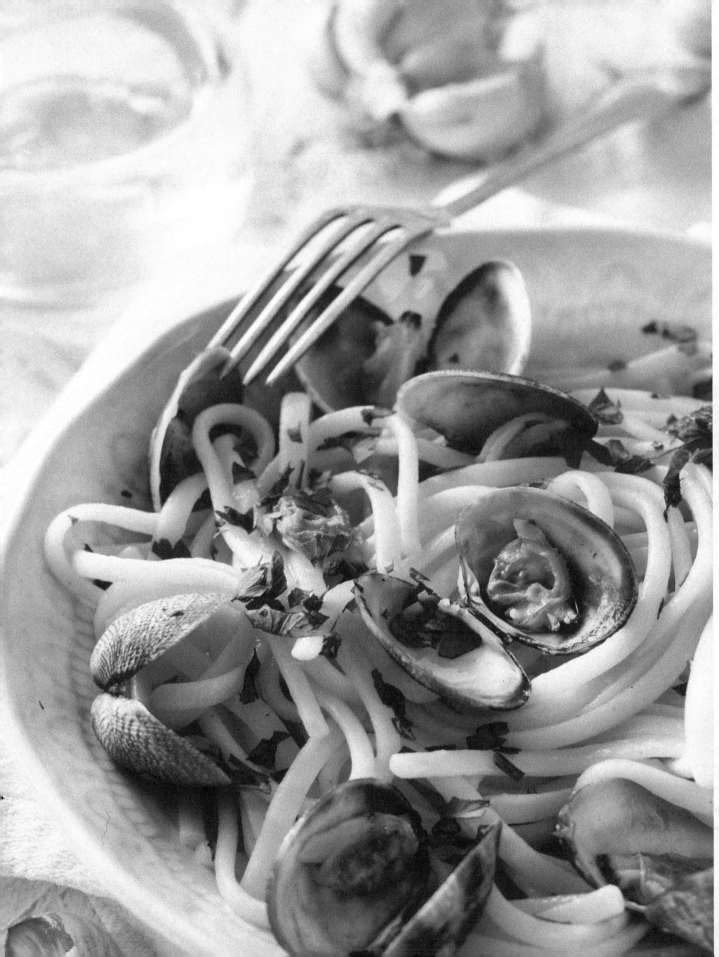

Bibliography

FROM THE SAME AUTHOR

ITALIAN COOKBOOK FOR ONE - More than 120 Very Easy Recipes for Beginners! Delight yourself like in a restaurant with the best meals for weight loss and heart health!

ITALIAN DIET FOR BEGINNERS *Cookbook* - 120+ Super Easy Recipes to Start a Healthier Lifestyle! Discover the tastiest Diet overall to lose weight and stay Healthy!

ITALIAN DIET FOR MEN *Cookbook* - More than 120 seafood, vegetarian and meat recipes from the Best Mediterranean Cuisine! Stay FIT and HEALTHY with the perfect diet to lose weight before summer!

ITALIAN DIET FOR WOMEN *Cookbook* - The Best 120+ recipes for weight loss and stay HEALTHY! Maintain FIT your body and delight yourself with the best diet overall for heart health!

ITALIAN DIET FOR KIDS *Cookbook* - The Most Delicious 120 Recipes for Children, tested BY Kids FOR Kids! Stay FIT and HEALTHY with many seafood and vegetarian meals, HAVING FUN as in a restaurant!

ITALIAN COOKBOOK FOR TWO - The Best 220+ Seafood and Vegetarian Recipes For Mum and Kids! Stay HEALTHY and lose weight preparing these delicious meals with your family!

ITALIAN COOKBOOK FOR COUPLE - 220+ Delicious Recipes to make together! Eat with your Partner as in a Restaurant with the most complete guide about the Italian Cuisine for two!

ITALIAN COOKBOOK FOR BEGINNER CHEF - More than 220 Very Easy Recipes to Start your Italian Restaurant Cuisine! Delight yourself and your Friends with the Best Mediterranean Meals like a Chef!

ITALIAN COOKBOOK FOR MEDITERRANEAN ATHLETES - The Best 220+ Seafood and Vegetarian Recipes For Weight Loss and Heart Health! Stay FIT and LIGHT with The Most Delicious Diet Overall!

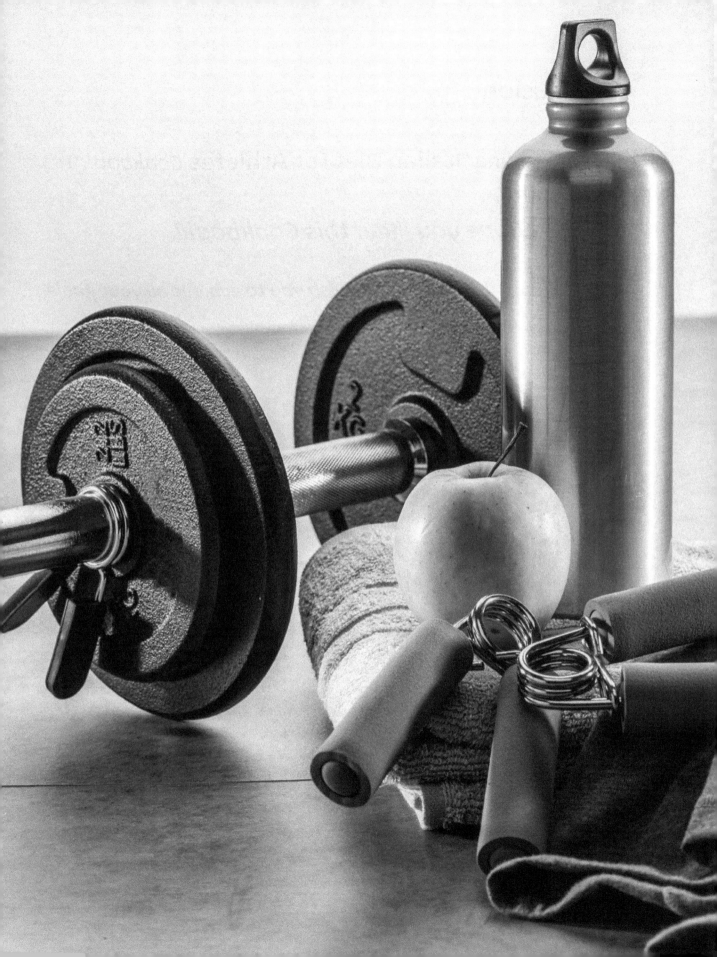

Conclusion

Thanks for reading "Italian Diet for Athletes *Cookbook*"!

I hope you liked this Cookbook!

I wish you to achieve all your goals!

Olivia Rossi

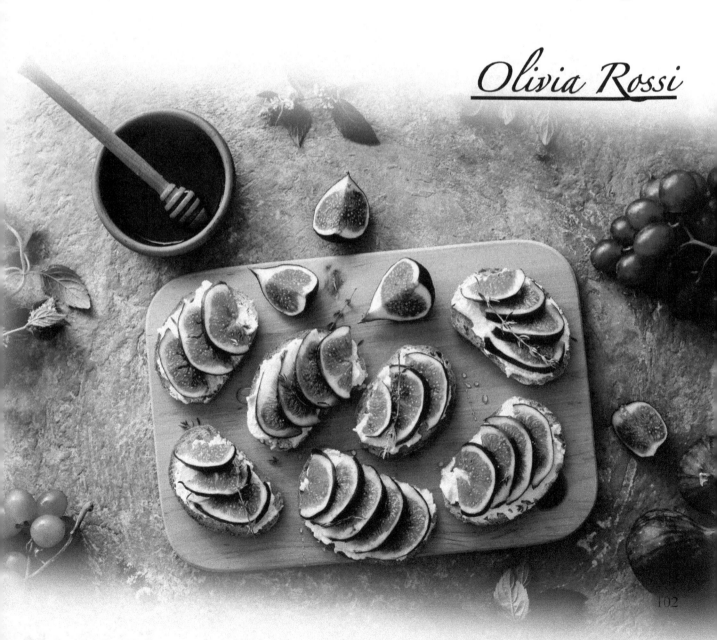

CPSIA information can be obtained
at www.ICGtesting.com
Printed in the USA
BVHW062126240521
607998BV00010B/1438